ATLAS OF LAPAROSCOPY AND HYSTEROSCOPY TECHNIQUES

Third Edition

Edited by

Togas Tulandi MD MHCM
Professor, Obstetrics and Gynecology, Milton Leong Chair in
Reproductive Medicine, McGill University,
Montreal, Canada

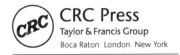

CRC Press
Taylor & Francis Group
Boca Raton London New York

CRC Press is an imprint of the
Taylor & Francis Group, an **informa** business

CRC Press
Taylor & Francis Group
6000 Broken Sound Parkway NW, Suite 300
Boca Raton, FL 33487-2742

First issued in paperback 2019

© 2007 by Taylor & Francis Group, LLC
CRC Press is an imprint of Taylor & Francis Group, an Informa business

No claim to original U.S. Government works

ISBN-13: 978-0-415-41440-1 (hbk)
ISBN-13: 978-0-367-38786-0 (pbk)

Visit the Taylor & Francis Web site at
http://www.taylorandfrancis.com

and the CRC Press Web site at
http://www.crcpress.com

To my family, colleagues, fellows, residents and operating room staff

Togas Tulandi

Contents

Contributors

Krisztina Ilona Bajzak
Gynecology and Laparoscopic Surgeons, PC,
Raleigh, NC
USA

Bulent Berker

Stefano Bettocchi
Associate Professor
DIGON (Department of Gynecology,
Obstetrics and Neonatology)
University of Bari
Italy

R Botchorishvili
CHU Bd Léon Malfreyt
Clermont Ferrand
France

Michel J Canis
Professor, CHU Bd Léon Malfreyt
Clermont Ferrand
France

Clementina Cantatore
DIGON (Department of Gynecology,
Obstetrics and Neonatology)
University of Bari
Italy

Oronzo Ceci
DiGON (Department of Gynecology,
Obstetrics and Neonatology)
University of Bari
Italy

Lynne Chapman
Clinical Research Fellow
Royal Free Hospital
London, UK

Aarathi Cholkeri-Singh
Newton-Wellestey Hospital
Minimally Invasive Gynecologic Unit
Newton, MA
USA

Luc De Catte
Fetal Medicine Unit
University Hospitals Leuven
Belgium

Jan Deprest
Professor, Fetal Medicine Unit
University Hospitals Leuven
Belgium

Roland Devlieger
Fetal Medicine Unit
University Hospitals Leuven
Belgium

Marie-Madeleine Dolmans
Catholic University of Louvain
Cliniques Universitaires St-Luc
Brussels, Belgium

Jacques Donnez
Catholic University of Louvain
Cliniques Universitaires St-Luc
Brussels, Belgium

Tatjana Dosev
Clinical Center, Beograd
Serbia

Sean Duffy
Senior Lecturer and Consultant Gynecologist
St James University Hospital
Leeds, UK

Alaa El-Ghobashy
Subspecialty Fellow in Gynecological Oncology
St James' University Hospital
Leeds, UK

Tommaso Falcone
Professor and Chairman
Cleveland Clinic Lerner College of Medicine
Case Western Reserve University
Cleveland
OH, USA

Stephan Gordts
Professor, Leuven Institute for Fertility and
Embryology
Leuven, Belgium

Roger Hart
Associate Professor Reproductive Medicine
University of Western Australia and
Medical Director of Fertility Specialists of
Perth, Western Australia

Keith Isaacson
Newton-Wellesley Hospital
Newton
MA, USA

Pascale Jadoul
Catholic University of Louvain
Cliniques Universitaires St-Luc
Brussels, Belgium

John M Jafettas

K Jardon
CHU Bd Léon Malfreyt
Clermont Ferrand
France

Philippe R Koninckx
University Hospital Gasthuisberg & Center for
Surgical Technologies
Catholic University Leuven
Belgium and John Radcliffe Hospital
University of Oxford
UK

Rose C Kung
Associate Professor, University of Toronto and
Sunnybrook and Women's Health Science Centre,
Toronto, ON
Canada

Anna Franca Laera
DiGON (Department of Gynecology,
Obstetrics and Neonatology)
University of Bari
Italy

Liesbeth Lewi
Fetal Medicine Unit
University Hospitals Leuven
Belgium

Moises Lichtinger
Holy Cross Hospital
Fort Lauderdale, FL
USA

Danielle E Luciano
Center for Fertility and Women's Health
New Britain General Hospital
New Britain, CT
USA

Anthony A Luciano
Center for Fertility and Women's Health,
New Britain General Hospital
New Britain, CT
USA

Thomas L Lyons
Center for Women's Care and Reproductive Surgery
Atlanta, GA
USA

H Manhes
CHU Bd Léon Malfreyt
Clermont Ferrand
France

G Mage
CHU Bd Léon Malfreyt
Clermont Ferrand
France

Adam Magos
Consultant Gynaecologist
University Department of Obstetrics and
Gynecology
Royal Free Hospital
London, UK

Suketu M Mansuria
Assistant Professor, University of Pittsburgh Medical
Center, Magee-Women's Hospital
Pittsburgh, PA
USA

Dan C Martin
Professor, University of Tennessee Health
Science Center
Memphis, TN
USA

Belen Martinez-Madrid
Catholic University of Louvain
Cliniques Universitaires St-Luc
Brussels, Belgium

Charles E Miller
Charles Miller and Associates
Chicago, IL
USA

Camran R Nezhat
Stanford University School of Medicine
Palo Alto, CA
USA

Ceana Nezhat
Mercer University School of Medicine
Atlanta, GA
USA

Farr R Nezhat
Director, Gynecologic Minimally Invasive Surgery
Mt Sinai School of Medicine
New York, NY
USA

Pui Shan NG
Associate Consulant and Honorary Clinical Assistant
Professor
Department of Obstetrics and Gynaecology
Prince of Wales Hospital
The Chinese University of Hong Kong,
Hong Kong

Mario Nutis

Jamie Ocampo

Peter O'Donovan
Professor, Bradford Royal Infirmary
Bradford
UK

Stefano Palomba
Professor, University Magna Graecia of Catanzaro
Catanzaro
Italy

Spyros Papaioannou
Consultant Obstetrician and Gynaecologist Princess
of Wales Women's Unit
Heartlands Hospital
Birmingham, UK

Sejal Dharia Patelc
Assistant Professor and Co-Director
The Ohio State University
Columbus, OH
USA

Marie Plante
Associate Professor
Department of Obstetric and Gynecology
Laval University
Gynecologic Oncologist
Centre Mospialiet Universitaire de Québec
L' Hôtel-Dieu de Québec
Quebec, Canada

Giovanni Pontrelli
DIGON (Department of Gynecology,
Obstetrics and Neonatology)
University of Bari
Italy

JL Pouly
CHU Bd Léon Malfreyt
Clermont Ferrand
France

B Rabischong
CHU Bd Léon Malfreyt
Clermont Ferrand
France

Lisa Marie Roberts
Gynecology and Laparoscopic Surgeons, PC
Raleigh, NC
USA

Michel Roy
Professor
Department of Obstetric and Gynecology
Laval University

Joseph S Sanfilippo
Professor and Vice Chairman
University of Pittsburgh Medical Center
Magee-Women's Hospital
Pittsburgh, PA
USA

Luigi Selvaggi
DIGON (Department of Gynecology,
Obstetrics and Neonatology)
University of Bari
Italy

Andrew A Shelton

Amudha Thangavelu
Clinical Research Fellow, St James' University
Hospital
Leeds, UK

Geoffrey Trew
Consultant in Reproductive Medicine and Surgery
Hammersmith and Queen Charlotte's Hospital
London, UK

Tim van Mieghem
Fetal Medicine Unit
University Hospitals Leuven
Belgium

Dominique van Schoubroeck
Fetal Medicine Unit
University Hospitals Leuven
Belgium

Pong Mo Yuen
Director of Minimally Invasive Gynaecology
Hong Kong Sanatorium and Hospital
Hong Kong Honorary Clinical Associate Professor
The Chinese University of Hong Kong
Hong Kong

Konstantin Zakashansky

Fulvio Zullo
Professor, University Magna Graecia of Catanzaro
Italy

Errico Zupi
University of Rome 'Tor Vergata'
Fatebenefratelli Hospital
Rome, Italy

Foreword

Telinde and Mattingly first recognized the importance of laparoscopy in the 4th edition of Operative Gynecology. They recognized the role of laparoscopy and culdoscopy for the diagnosis of ectopic pregnancy but forecasted that the new technique (laparoscopy) would gain wide spread acceptance because of positional advantage and a wider range of visibility of the entire peritoneal cavity. Since this statement regarding the future, laparoscopy has achieved a prominent position in the field of gynecologic surgery. Most pelvic surgery performed by laparotomy may now be performed either completely with or assisted with the laparoscope. Moreover, the hysteroscope has attained an indispensable role in the diagnosis and treatment of uterine pathology.

The third edition of The Atlas of Laparascopy and Hysteroscopic Techniques for the Gynecologist presents the advances of the field since the last edition published in 1999. The chapters assembled and edited by Professor Tulandi represent the World's leading experts in the field who possess an intimate knowledge of the specialty coupled with an extensive experience in the operating room. The illustrations are excellent. The discussions are concise, concrete, and thorough. The text presents a worldwide view of the advances in the field. This edition is a superb addition to the medical literature and will serve as a welcome reference for the gynecologic surgeon.

John A Rock
Senior Vice President, Medical Affairs
Dean, College of Medicine
Professor Obstetrics and Gynecology
Florida International University
University Park, Miami, Florida, USA

Preface

The second edition of *Atlas of Laparoscopy and Hysteroscopy Techniques* has proven popular among gynecologists, residents, and fellows-in-training. The format is well liked by readers; most are busy practicing gynecologists who want to learn step-by-step techniques of a surgical procedure. With the advances in endoscopic technique and the invention of newer equipment and instruments, there is an urgent need to update the book. Among relatively new techniques are robotic surgery, transvaginal hydrolaparoscopy, laparoscopic radical hysterectomy, laparoscopic abdominal cerclage, and hysteroscopic sterilization.

As many gynecologists become more familiar with and start performing different types of laparoscopic hysterectomy, we have divided the discussion into laparoscopic supracervical hysterectomy, total hysterectomy, and radical hysterectomy. On the other hand, salpingoscopy and falloposcopy are rarely performed now, and these subjects have been dropped from this edition. In this edition, we have added chapters on management and prevention of laparoscopic and hysteroscopic complications.

The contributors are gynecologic surgeons who are acknowledged leaders in gynecologic endoscopic surgery with many years of experience. The first three chapters discuss basic principles of advanced laparoscopy. The following 21 chapters are dedicated to laparoscopic procedures, including hysterectomies, abdominal cerclage, laparoscopy in pediatrics and adolescents, and transvaginal hydrolaparoscopy. These chapters are followed by a discussion of endoscopic fetal surgery and nine chapters on hysteroscopy technique and procedures. The final two chapters deal with complications of laparoscopy and hysteroscopic surgery.

This is a manual for practicing gynecologists, residents, and fellows-in-training. Readers will gain an understanding of the practical step-by-step techniques involved in laparoscopic and hysteroscopic procedures and will learn about the potential complications and how to avoid them. As in the previous editions, we maintain the simple and easy-to read format of the book.

Togas Tulandi

Basic principles of laparoscopic surgery

Togas Tulandi

Advances in technology, including instrumentation and video-imaging, have led to rapid progress in laparoscopic surgery. Accordingly, we can perform many procedures that previously required a laparotomy by laparoscopy. Operative laparoscopy, however, demands a higher degree of technical skill and a greater variety of equipment than required for diagnostic laparoscopy or tubal sterilization. Knowledge of anatomy and pathology and the familiarity of the surgeon with the instruments are mandatory. Depending upon personal preference, the surgeon can perform the procedure using laser, ultrasound scalpel, electrocautery, or scissors.

SETUP

The setup should ideally involve at least two video monitor screens (Figures 1.1 and 1.2). The surgeon stands facing one monitor on the opposite side, with the assistant facing the second monitor. The second assistant, if needed, stands or sits at the end of the table, between the patient's legs. For a setup with just one video monitor, the monitor is placed at the end of the operating table between the patient's legs, for easy viewing by both the surgeon and the assistant (Figure 1.3). A surgical team familiar with operative laparoscopy is invaluable. They are responsible for the operation of electrosurgical generators, lasers, and suction irrigators. They should be knowledgeable with regard of all laparoscopic instruments and should know how to find a backup instrument at short notice.

POSITIONING AND PREPARATION

In the lithotomy position, the patient is placed horizontally until insertion of the laparoscope into the abdominal cavity. Instead of Candy Cane stirrups, we recommend the use of Allen-type stirrups, where padding supports and protects the calf and foot. Protection of the lateral aspect of the knee prevents peroneal nerve compression. In addition, abduction and adduction are performed at the handle, and this could be done during the procedure if needed. The thighs are placed almost parallel to the abdomen (Figure 1.4). This will facilitate manipulation of instruments. A rigid intrauterine cannula is inserted into the uterus to allow manipulation of the uterus and to permit chromopertubation. We prefer a disposable plastic intrauterine cannula (Humi syringe).

An intravenous line is inserted through the patient's arm on the assistant's side, and the arm on the side of the operating surgeon should be placed by the patient's side and protected with an ulnar pad. An extended arm will interfere with the surgeon's mobility. Furthermore, brachial plexus neuropathy has been reported after laparoscopic surgery using a steep Trendelenburg position with shoulder braces and the patient's arm extended at 90°.

To ensure that the bladder is empty throughout the procedure, an indwelling catheter is left inside the bladder and removed at the end of the operation. When extensive adhesion or advanced endometriosis requiring dissection near the bowel is anticipated, bowel prep is indicated. Simple bowel prep is obtained by drinking 90 ml of phospha-soda

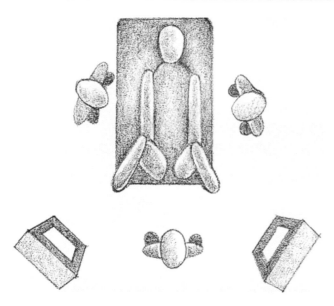

Figure 1.1 Operating room setup for two video monitors. The surgeon stands facing one monitor on the opposite side and the assistant faces the second monitor. The second assistant, if needed, stands or sits at the end of the table, between the patient's legs.

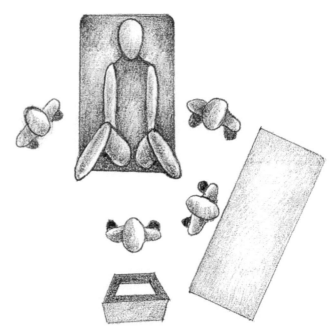

Figure 1.3 Operating room setup for single video monitor. The monitor is placed at the end of the operating table between the patient's legs, for easy viewing by both the surgeon and the assistant.

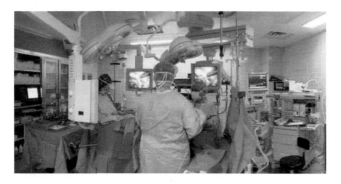

Figure 1.2 Operating room setup for three video monitors.

solution the day before surgery. Shaving of the abdomen and pubic area is not required. Laparoscopy of the pelvic organs is done in the Trendelenburg position (about 30°).

TROCAR INSERTION

The primary trocar is inserted via a 1 cm infraumbilical incision. The type of incision (horizontal or vertical) depends on the configuration of the umbilicus. Direct trocar insertion without the use of a Veress needle can be done using a disposable trocar. It has a retractable inner trocar, and its tip is always sharp. We prefer to create a pneumoperitoneum before inserting

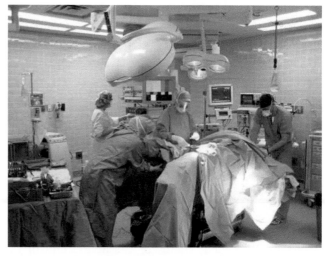

Figure 1.4 Preparation for laparoscopic surgery. Note that the patient's thighs are placed almost parallel to the abdomen, facilitating manipulation of the laparoscopic instruments. The arm is tucked beside the body.

the trocar. In nonobese women, a Veress needle or primary trocar is inserted at 45° from the horizontal (Figure 1.5). The aortic bifurcation in nonobese women is located about 0.4 cm cranial to the umbilicus. In obese women, the bifurcation is approximately 2.5 cm cranial to the umbilicus, and so the angle of

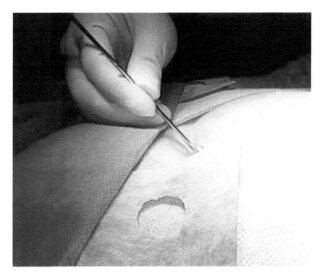

Figure 1.5 Insertion of a Veress needle. In a thin woman, we hold the needle a few centimeters from its tip.

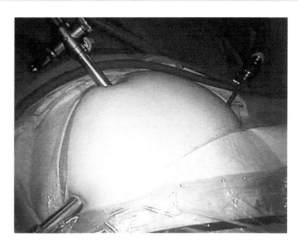

Figure 1.6 Sites of trocars.

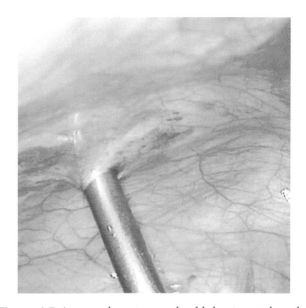

Figure 1.7 A secondary trocar should be inserted under laparoscopic control, lateral to the deep epigastric vessels.

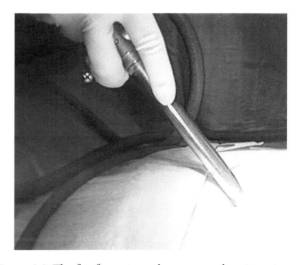

Figure 1.8 The forefinger is used to prevent deep insertion.

insertion can be safely increased. In patients who have undergone multiple laparotomies, an open laparoscopy using a blunt trocar is recommended. A trocar sleeve loaded with a laparoscope is an alternative to a blunt trocar.

Pneumoperitoneum is achieved by insufflating the abdominal cavity with carbon dioxide (CO_2) gas. The gas is infused at a rate of 1–3 liters/min, and the intraabdominal pressure should be below 20 mmHg. The abdomen is observed for global distension and the disappearance of liver dullness. Adequate pneumoperitoneum is usually obtained with 2–3 liters of CO_2. After insertion of the laparoscope, the abdominal cavity should first be evaluated for possible inadvertent injury by the Veress needle or trocar.

We routinely use two secondary 5 mm trocars. Depending on the type of surgery, these are usually inserted just above the pubic hairline, lateral to the deep epigastric vessels (Figure 1.6). For removal of a large mass such as an ovarian cyst or uterine myoma, we place the secondary trocars higher than the upper pole of the mass. If removal of a specimen via the trocar is anticipated, one of the lateral trocars should be 10 mm. The trocars should always be inserted under direct laparoscopic control (Figure 1.7). We recommend the use of a forefinger as a guard to prevent too deep insertion (Figure 1.8).

An incisional hernia may occur if the incision is $\geq$ 10 mm. A deep suture with 2-0 polyglycolic acid suture to approximate the fascia is required. This is particularly needed for a nonmidline incision.

Examination of abdominal organs

The abdominal and pelvic organs should be thoroughly examined. Occasionally, the view to the pelvic organs is obstructed due to the presence of adhesions to the anterior abdominal wall (Figure 1.9a). In this case, the laparoscope is introduced into the secondary trocar and lysis of adhesions is performed using scissors inserted through the primary umbilical trocar, or the opposite secondary trocar (Figure 1.9b). An obstructed view of the entire abdominal cavity is now obtained (Figures 1.10–1.12).

UNDERWATER INSPECTION

Near the completion of a laparoscopic procedure, irrigation of the abdominal cavity should be performed. Complete hemostasis is mandatory. Peritoneal lavage is reformed until the irrigating solution is free from blood and debris. The pneumoperitoneum acts as a temporary tamponade, and bleeding may occur after the gas is evacuated from the abdominal cavity. Inspection of the operative field after instillation of approximately 500–1000 ml of Ringer's lactate or

(a)

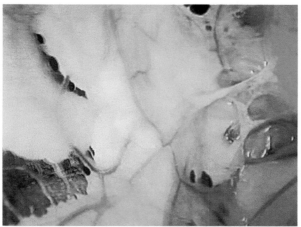

(b)

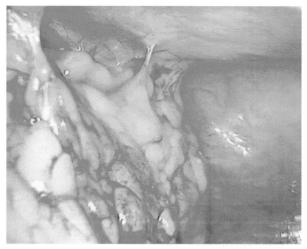

Figure 1.9 (a) The view of the pelvic organs is obstructed due to the presence of severe and dense adhesions to the anterior abdominal wall. (b) In this case, the laparoscope is introduced into the secondary trocar, and lysis of adhesions is performed.

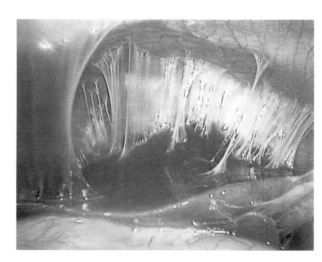

Figure 1.10 The abdominal cavity, including the upper abdomen, should be systemically inspected. Here, perihepatic adhesions are seen.

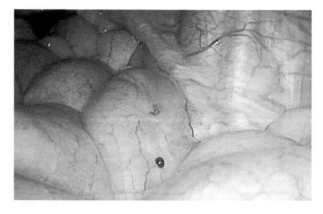

Figure 1.11 Endometriosis on the intestine.

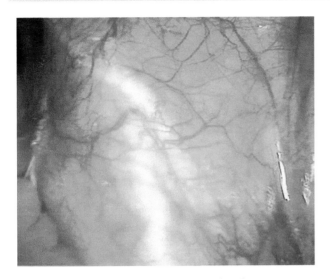

Figure 1.12 View of the ureter on the pelvic brim.

normal saline ('examination underwater') allows identification of bleeding points.

ANESTHESIA

For operative laparoscopy, general anesthesia with endotracheal intubation is mandatory. Before intubation, one should avoid assisting ventilation with the use of a mask, which may inflate the stomach. Otherwise, a nasogastric tube should be inserted to deflate the stomach before insertion of a Veress needle or a trocar. Adequate ventilation is mandatory during the laparoscopic procedure. Rapid absorption of CO_2 gas and decrease of lung expansion due to the pneumoperitoneum and Trendelenburg position may result in hypercarbia. Cardiac arrhythmias may then occur. If vasopressin is used, the surgeon should notify the anesthetist before its administration. Although rare, its use has been associated with cardiac arrhythmia and pulmonary edema.

COMPLICATIONS AND PREVENTION OF INJURY TO DEEP EPIGASTRIC VESSELS

Injury to the deep epigastric vessels is avoided by transillumination of the abdominal wall before trocar insertion and by visualization of the vessels on the peritoneal surface of the anterior abdomen by the laparoscope. The vessels, which are located lateral to the obliterated umbilical artery, should be avoided. Despite these measures, occasionally a large vessel is injured and brisk bleeding occurs. This can be controlled by a figure-of-eight suture with a retention suture. Under direct laparoscopic control, a large needle is placed through the whole thickness of the abdominal wall with the trocar in situ. The trocar is then removed and the suture is tied.

An alternative is to use a Foley catheter. A # 16 catheter is first inserted into the abdominal cavity via the trocar. The balloon is inflated to 30 ml, the trocar is removed, and the catheter is retracted outside until the balloon is tightly compressing the bleeding site. A clamp is placed on the outer side of the catheter at skin level to maintain traction and hemostasis. The suture and the catheter can be removed after 24 hours.

SUGGESTED READING

- Hurd WH, Bude RO, DeLancey JOL, Pearl ML. The relationship of the umbilicus to the aortic bifurcation: Implications for laparoscopic technique. Obstet Gynecol 1992;80:48–51.
- Tulandi T, Bugnah M. Operative laparoscopy: surgical modalities. Fertil Steril 1995;63:237–45.
- Tulandi T, Beique F, Kimia M. Pulmonary edema: a complication of local injection of vasopressin at laparoscopy. Fertil Steril 1996;66:478–80.

2

Laparoscopic instrumentation

Lisa M Roberts and Krisztina Bajzak

INSTRUMENTATION FOR VISUALIZATION

Compared with laparotomy, the primary advantage of laparoscopic surgery is good visualization of the entire abdominal cavity. An image is dispatched through a telescope to a camera, then a video processor unit, and finally to the monitor or other imaging screen. This transmission must occur using a high-quality light source and light cable.

Monitor

The horizontal resolution of a monitor is measured in lines, and is typically 400–700 lines. The resolution of the monitor should exceed that of the camera so that the monitor does not diminish the quality of the image.

Camera

Camera heads (Figure 2.1), typically attached to the eyepiece of the scope, may come separately or as one unit. The camera heads house charge-coupled devices (CCDs) that take an image at the eyepiece and electronically convert it to a digitized image that is received by the video processor. The video processor then transmits the image to the video monitor, printer, CD/DVD burner, and/or memory stick. The image quality is significantly dependent upon the lines of resolution.

CCDs are available as single-chip and three-chip devices. Single-chip cameras deliver 400–450 lines of resolution, whereas three-chip cameras deliver over 700 lines. In addition, three-chip cameras have a prism system to separate colors (red, green, and blue) and increase resolution, producing a sharper image. The practical lifespan of a camera is 2–3 years before it becomes technologically obsolete.

Light source

Most laparoscopists prefer to use a 300 W xenon light source (Figure 2.2) because it has a color temperature of 5600 K, equivalent to the sun, and produces a more natural color spectrum. Alternatively, a halide light source is available, but this tends to produce a bluish tint.

Light cable transmitter

In addition to the light source, the image quality is dependent on the cable that transmits the light from the source to the camera. Light cables are available with fiber bundles or fluid. Fluid-filled cables transmit light better than fibers, but may not be autoclaved and are more rigid and heavier. Fiber cables should be handled with care, since multiple broken fibers will decrease the amount of transmitted light and decrease the quality of the image.

Care must be taken not to allow the distal end of the active light cable to rest on the surgical drape or the patient. The tip of the cable may become very hot, and can cause a fire on the drape or a skin burn.

Telescope

The final device critical to a high-quality image is the laparoscope itself (Figure 2.3). An image starts at the

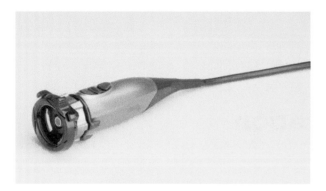

Figure 2.1 Camera. (© Karl Storz Endoscopy-America, Inc.)

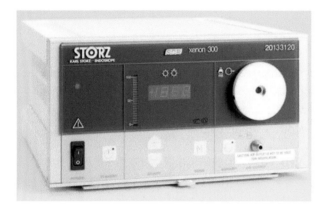

Figure 2.2 Light source. (© Karl Storz Endoscopy-America, Inc.)

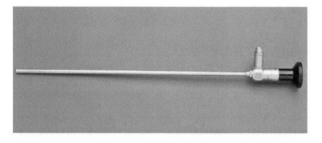

Figure 2.3 Telescope. (© Karl Storz Endoscopy-America, Inc.)

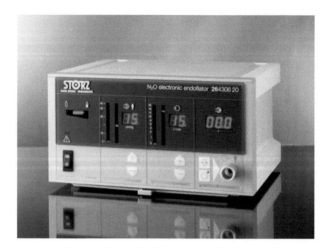

Figure 2.4 Insufflator. (© Karl Storz Endoscopy-America, Inc.)

have an operating channel through which instruments can be inserted.

Insufflator

An insufflation unit (Figure 2.4) will allow the operator to control the rate of carbon dioxide (CO_2) flow and the maximum pressure of the pneumoperitoneum. Certain units offer a heating feature that will warm and humidify the CO_2 gas as it flows into the abdomen. This feature is useful especially when frequent or voluminous irrigation is performed with solution that is not warmed above room temperature.

A laparoscopic tower (Figure 2.5) or boom suspended from the ceiling will hold a monitor, video processor, light source, and gas insufflators.

ACCESS INSTRUMENTS

Access to the abdominal cavity may be achieved using an open or closed approach. An open approach is performed by making a small incision through all layers of the abdominal wall until the peritoneal cavity is entered, usually at the base of the umbilicus. Then, a blunt-tipped canulla (Figure 2.6) is inserted through the incision and secured in place using fascial sutures. A closed entry may be performed with or without insufflation.

A Veress needle (Figure 2.7) is passed through a small skin incision directly into the peritoneal cavity, and CO_2 is insufflated through this needle. Once the

lens of the scope and is adversely affected by chips or cracks on the lens cover. It is helpful to warm the distal tip of the laparoscope prior to insertion into the peritoneal cavity, since otherwise fogging may occur. Laparoscopes are available in 0°, 30°, 45°, and 70° angles. A wide angle allows greater light absorption, which must be compensated by the light source and the camera. Laparoscopes are available in 2–11 mm diameters. Most gynecologists operate with a 0°, 5 mm or 10 mm laparoscope. Larger-diameter scopes may

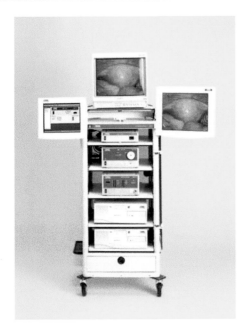

Figure 2.5 Laparoscopic tower. (© Karl Storz Endoscopy-America, Inc.)

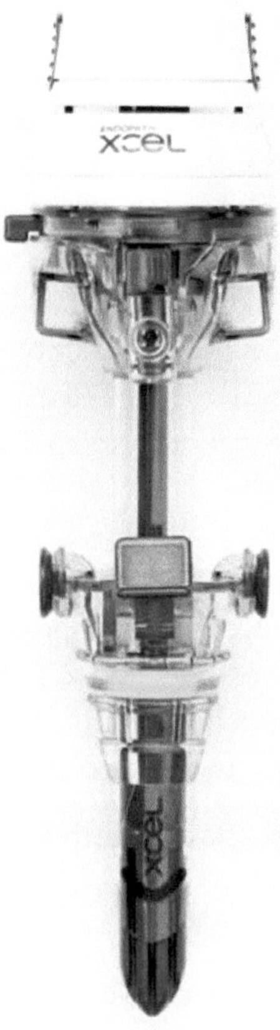

pneumoperitoneum has been established and the desired intraabdominal pressure has been reached, the surgeon inserts a trocar through the skin incision, either blindly or under visualization (Figure 2.8).

Trocars are available as disposable plastic (Figures 2.9 and 2.10) or reusable steel (Figure 2.11). If steel trocars are used, it is important to keep the inner trocar sharp for easy insertion. Trocars are also available in different sizes, ranging from 2 or 12 mm, and are selected based on the anticipated use of the operating instruments.

OPERATING INSTRUMENTS

Graspers

Graspers vary greatly in the design of their tips. Atraumatic graspers (Figure 2.12) allow the surgeon to

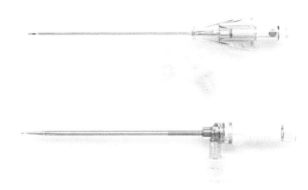

Figure 2.7 Insufflation needles. (Courtesy of Ethicon Endo-Surgery, Inc. All rights reserved.)

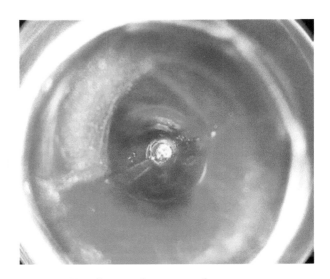

Figure 2.8 Visualization during cannula insertion.

Figure 2.6 Blunt-tipped cannula. (Courtesy of Ethicon Endo-Surgery, Inc. All rights reserved.)

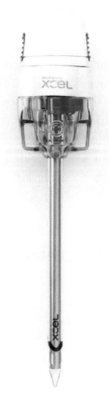

Figure 2.9 Bladeless trocar and cannula. (Courtesy of Ethicon Endo-Surgery, Inc. All rights reserved.)

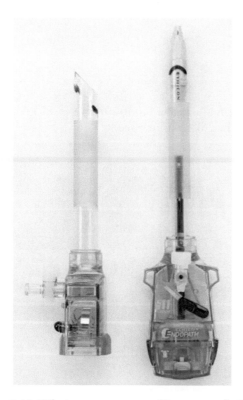

Figure 2.10 Dilating tip trocar. (Courtesy of Ethicon Endo-Surgery, Inc. All rights reserved.)

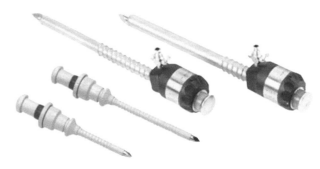

Figure 2.11 Reusable trocars. (Wolf.)

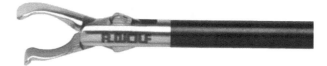

Figure 2.12 Atraumatic grasper. (Wolf.)

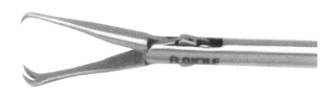

Figure 2.13 Tenaculum grasper. (Wolf.)

handle delicate tissue such as a fallopian tube or ureter, whereas traumatic graspers (Figure 2.13) offer better holding ability, and are helpful for tissue removal. The grasper handles may be locking or nonlocking. A corkscrew and single-tooth tenaculum offer secure tissue holding ability, and are especially helpful in removal of less vascular organs such as during myomectomy or hysterectomy.

Scissors

Laparoscopic scissors also vary greatly in their design. Scissors may be reusable or disposable. Their tips may be pointed (Figures 2.14 and 2.15), blunt, or hooked (Figure 2.16). Attached monopolar or bipolar energy offers the capacity to cut or coagulate.

Electrosurgical Instruments

Bipolar energy

In our standard practice, we do not start any laparoscopic procedure until an electrosurgical instrument for achieving hemostasis is available and has been tested to confirm that it is in working condition.

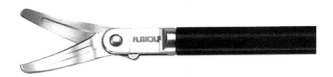

Figure 2.14 Curved scissors. (© Karl Storz Endoscopy-America, Inc.)

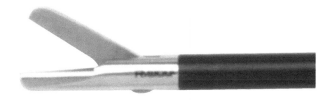

Figure 2.15 Adhesiolysis scissors. (Wolf.)

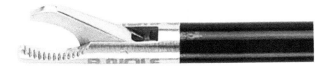

Figure 2.16 Hooked scissors. (Wolf.)

Many devices are available, and are selected based on the surgeon's preference. Bipolar energy is most effective for hemostasis. It works by conducting electrical current between the jaws of the forceps. The Kleppinger forceps (Figure 2.17) has been the standard bipolar device for many years. Newer bipolar devices have limited lateral thermal spread, lower contact temperatures, and greater mechanical compressive forces. In addition, some offer a concomitant tissue cutting ability.

Monopolar energy

Monopolar electrosurgical devices are often used to cut tissue, and sometimes for hemostasis. The electrical current is transferred through the device, and continued through the tissue until it finds the return electrode – often a pad located on the patient's thigh. Compared with bipolar devices, they are associated with greater risk of injury, since the electrical pathway is longer, and presents an opportunity for direct or capacitive coupling.

Harmonic Scalpel

The Harmonic Scalpel (Ethicon Endo-Surgery, Inc., Cincinnati, OH) (Figure 2.18) uses mechanical energy to cut and coagulate tissue and vessels.

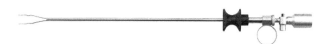

Figure 2.17 Kleppinger bipolar forceps. (Wolf.)

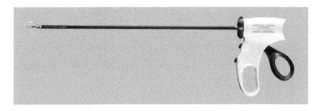

Figure 2.18 Harmonic Scalpel. (Courtesy of Ethicon Endo-Surgery, Inc. All rights reserved.)

It converts electrical energy into mechanical motion, resulting in vibration of an active blade at a rate of 55 500 Hz. An inactive blade acts as a backstop. This vibration causes the proteins of the intervening tissue to denature and creates a protein coagulum that seals smaller vessels. The mechanical secondary heat seals larger vessels. This process is performed at a relatively low temperature (50–100°C), reducing lateral thermal spread to surrounding tissues.

Lasers

Surgical lasers are also used in operative laparoscopy. Over the years, the use of lasers has become less common. This is due to the high efficacy and low cost of electrosurgical devices. The most common lasers used in gynecology are the CO_2, neodymium: yttrium aluminum garnet (Nd:YAG), and argon– potassium titanyl phosphate (KTP) lasers. The CO_2 laser is usually used with irrigation fluid as a backstop to minimize the depth of penetration during cutting or vaporization. The thermal spread is limited to approximately 0.1 mm.

The articulated arm of the CO_2 laser is attached to an operating laparoscope using a direct coupler that houses a mirror and focusing lens. The lens and mirror focus and align the beam that passes through the operating channel. The CO_2 insufflation tubing is attached to the operating channel distal to the mirror to allow flow of CO_2 down the channel, minimizing smoke accumulation. The presence of smoke or fogging of the mirror or lens reduces the power density of the beam.

The Nd:YAG and KTP lasers are contact lasers, transmitting energy along a fiber. This can be used through ancillary trocars or the operating channel of the laparoscope. The KTP laser works well to cut and coagulate tissue. As the tip of the fiber approaches the tissue, the power density increases and the laser is used for cutting. As the tip is moved away from the tissue, the spot size increases and the power density decreases. The Nd:YAG laser coagulates well, but does not cut well unless a sapphire tip is used to increase the power density.

Smoke evacuator

Tissue ablation using electrocautery is associated with smoke formation, decreasing visualization. This can be minimized by using an effective smoke evacuator.

Suction–Irrigator

A suction and irrigation device is necessary in laparoscopic procedures where bleeding is anticipated. An irrigation device may be as simple as injecting irrigation fluid through a hollow blunt probe and aspirating using a syringe. We prefer a high-flow suction–irrigator. This is effective in situations with moderate or large amounts of bleeding.

Morcellator

Morcellators (Figure 2.19) offer efficient removal of large volumes of tissue through small incisions – typically 12–20 mm. It is important that the surgeon be properly trained to use a morcellator. It could lead to serious damage to surrounding organs or fatal hemorrhage. The original manual morcellator has been replaced by faster electromechanical morcellators. They are available as disposable or reusable devices.

Staplers

Laparoscopic staplers (Figure 2.20) seal blood vessels and cut tissue simultaneously. Depending on tissue thickness, a cartridge of variable length is inserted into the stapler device, and applied across the tissue. The diameter of the shaft is usually 12 mm. Six rows of staples compress the tissue and a blade cuts through the middle two rows, resulting in tissue separation with three rows of staples on each side.

Vascular clips

Endoclips (Figure 2.21) are useful for achieving hemostasis if the bleeding vessel can be visualized and

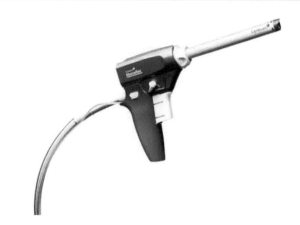

Figure 2.19 Morcellator: Gynecare Morcellex. (Reproduced with permission from ETHICON, INC., 2006 Somerville, NJ.)

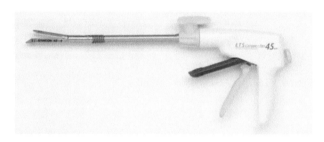

Figure 2.20 Staplers. (Courtesy of Ethicon Endo-Surgery, Inc. All rights reserved.)

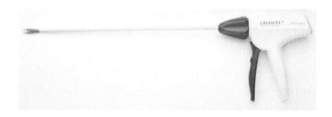

Figure 2.21 Endoclips. (Courtesy of Ethicon Endo-Surgery, Inc. All rights reserved.)

is located adjacent to tissue or structures where thermal injury from an electrosurgical device is a concern. A 6 mm × 1.2 mm stainless steel clip loaded onto an application device is used to grasp, compress, and secure a bleeding vessel.

Endoscopic loop

An endoscopic loop (Figure 2.22) is useful for ligating pedicles or organs, such as in oophorectomy, salpingectomy, and appendectomy procedures. A suture loop with a slipknot is introduced, together with an applicator, through a 5 mm cannula. Typically, three loops are placed, followed by transection of the organ.

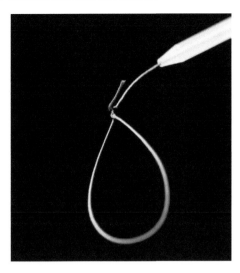

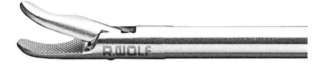

Figure 2.23 Curved needle holder. (Wolf.)

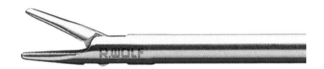

Figure 2.24 Straight needle holder. (Wolf.)

Figure 2.22 Endoscopic loop: Endoloop. (Courtesy of Ethicon Endo-Surgery, Inc. All rights reserved.)

Suturing instruments

Laparoscopic suturing is the most advanced skill of a laparoscopic surgeon. Needle holders are available with curved (Figure 2.23) or straight (Figure 2.24) tips, and may be self-righting. They should have a secure locking mechanism to keep the needle from rotating during tissue insertion. Sutures with straight or curved needles can be used through a 5 mm trocar sleeve. The knot is secured either with an intracorporeal suture tie or extracorporeally using a knot pusher.

The Endo Stitch (Tyco Healthcare, Mansfield, MA) (Figure 2.25) is a disposable 10 mm suturing device that has two jaws. A single-use needle and suture is loaded onto a jaw and passed through the tissue to the other jaw by closing the handles and flipping the toggle levers. It may be used to place interrupted or running stitches. LSI Solutions (Victor, NY) has a similar 5 mm suturing device.

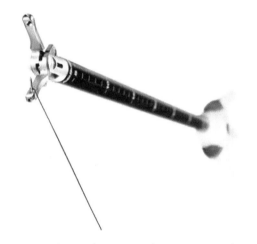

Figure 2.25 Endo Stitch suturing device. (Copyright © 2006 United States Surgical, a division of Tyco Healthcare Group LP. All rights reserved. Reprinted with the Permission of United States Surgical, a division of Tyco Healthcare Group LP.)

Specimen retrieval bags

Specimen retrieval bags (Figure 2.26) are useful to remove tissue without rupturing its contents within the peritoneal cavity (e.g., ovarian cysts) or without making contact with the layers of the abdominal wall (e.g., infectious tissue and endometriosis), or to facilitate efficient removal of multiple specimens (e.g., myomas). The bags come in a variety of sizes, shapes, and materials. Some bags may be rolled, inserted through a trocar sleeve, then opened using graspers, and closed by pulling on strings closing the mouth of

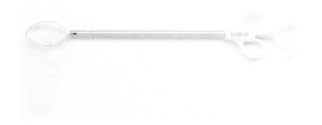

Figure 2.26 Specimen retrieval bag. (Courtesy of Ethicon Endo-Surgery, Inc. All rights reserved.)

the bag. We prefer a pouch with a metal ring around its mouth facilitating opening and closing of the bag.

Uterine manipulators

Uterine manipulators assist mobilization of the uterus. They are available as reusable or disposable devices, with or without tubing for chromopertubation.

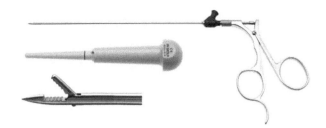

Figure 2.27 Fascial closure forceps and guide. (Wolf.)

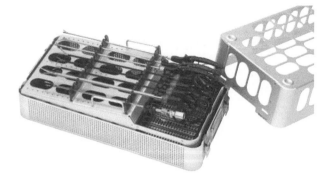

Figure 2.28 Laparoscopy tray. (Wolf.)

Many have a locking mechanism, freeing the surgeon's hand or at least decreasing fatigue. A simple method of creating a uterine manipulator is to place a single-tooth tenaculum on the anterior cervix and a cervical dilator into the uterine cavity, then to Steri-Strip the two together.

Hand-access device for hand-assisted laparoscopy

Hand-assisted laparoscopy using a hand-access device allows the surgeon to place the nondominant hand in the abdominal cavity and use conventional laparoscopy instruments in the dominant hand. This method combines tactile sensation, tissue palpation, retraction, blunt dissection, and spatial orientation similar to open surgery. It facilitates laparoscopic surgery, especially for the beginner.

Wound closure system

Full-thickness closure for laparoscopic incisions should be performed if the defect is ≥ 10 mm. In patients with a thick abdominal wall, full-thickness closure may be difficult resulting in an increased risk for incisional hernia formation. A wound closure system (Figure 2.27) consists of a needle passer that introduces a suture through the fascia. The suture is dropped and grasped on the opposite side with the same needle passer, and then withdrawn to allow for tight closure of the fascial layer and prevention of hernia formation.

LAPAROSCOPIC SET

When selecting instruments for a laparoscopic set, the skill of the surgeon and the anticipated procedures to be performed should be taken into consideration. The following is suggested as a guideline.

Standard laparoscopy tray

This should include (Figure 2.28):

- telescopes (0°, 30° 5 mm, 10 mm, operating)
- trocars
- bipolar forceps
- atraumatic grasping forceps
- traumatic grasping forceps (biopsy, Allis, or Adson forceps)
- blunt probe
- scissors (blunt and pointed)
- cyst aspiration needle
- suction/irrigator
- uterine manipulator

Advanced laparoscopy set

This should also include:

- corkscrew
- single-tooth tenaculum
- needle holders
- knot pusher
- rectal probe

Stand-by instruments

- morcellator
- Harmonic Scalpel
- endoscopic vascular clips
- endoscopic suture loop
- specimen retrieval bags
- wound closure device
- smoke evacuator
- hand-access device

3

Laparoscopic suturing

Togas Tulandi

All advanced laparoscopic surgeons should be able to perform laparoscopic suturing. This is a necessary skill for successful performance of a variety of laparoscopic procedures. An endoscopic loop, surgical staples, or clips cannot replace suturing. Sutures approximate tissue planes and establish hemostasis. Surgeons should acquire this important skill. Unexpected situations, including bleeding, uterine perforation, and bladder or intestinal tears, can be sutured laparoscopically, sparing the patient from a laparotomy.

Surgeons can perform suturing with intracorporeal or extracorporeal knot-tying, using different types and sizes of needles and suture materials. Most laparoscopic surgeons suture with intracorporeal knot-tying. For laparoscopic suturing, we use a 10 mm trocar with a reducer. The length of the suture depends on the type of suturing. For a single or a figure-of-eight suture, the suture length is about 10 cm, whereas for a continuous suture, 15–20 cm length is appropriate (Figure 3.1). There are several types of laparoscopic needle-drivers (see Chapter 2). Use a universal needle-driver with a ratchet; its jaw should be secure without bending a fine needle.

INTRACORPOREAL KNOT-TYING

- After many years of performing laparoscopic suturing, my preference is to use a ski-needle and intracorporeal knot-tying.
- For sutures thicker than 2.0, one has to create one's own ski-needle. This is done by bending a curved needle with two standard needle-drivers

normally used for laparotomies. The use of a ski-needle facilitates insertion of the needle into the abdominal cavity.

- The suture is held with a needle-driver at its midpoint and is inserted into a 10 mm reducer. The loaded needle-driver inside the reducer is readvanced through the trocar into the abdominal cavity.
- Those surgeons who prefer or use a 5 mm trocar, should take the following steps:
  - Grasp the end of the suture in the needle-driver jaws.
  - Withdraw the needle-driver through the reducer, letting the suture needle float freely beyond the end of the introducer (Figure 3.2).
  - Release the suture from the jaws of the needle-driver outside the reducer.
  - Reintroduce the needle-driver into the introducer.
  - Grasp the suture with the needle-driver a few centimeters from the needle, keeping the needle curve parallel to the driver and the reducer.
  - Pull the suture taut; withdraw the loaded needle-driver into the reducer until the entire suture needle is inside the distal end.
  - The loaded needle-driver inside the reducer is readvanced through the trocar into the abdominal cavity (Figure 3.2) until the surgeon can see the entire suture.
- The needle is grasped with the needle-driver, and the tissue is sutured. Proper placement of the

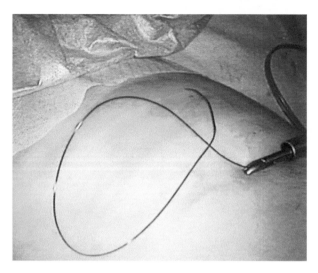

Figure 3.1 The length of the suture depends on the type of suturing.

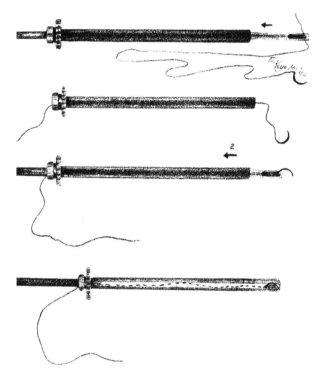

Figure 3.2 The end of the suture is grasped with a needle-driver and then withdrawn into the reducer until it is completely outside the introducer. The needle-driver is reinserted into the introducer (1) and the needle is positioned to allow withdrawal of the loaded needle-driver into the introducer (2). The loaded introducer can now be inserted into the abdominal cavity, and is ready to be used.

needle in the needle-driver can be challenging. We use the uterus or other organs to place the needle and re-grasp the needle until proper placement is achieved (Figure 3.3).

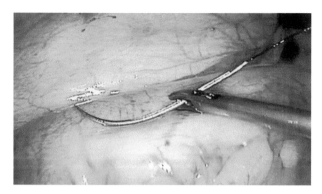

Figure 3.3 Proper placement of the needle in the needle-driver can be challenging. The uterus or other organs can be used to place the needle, which is then re-grasped until proper placement is achieved.

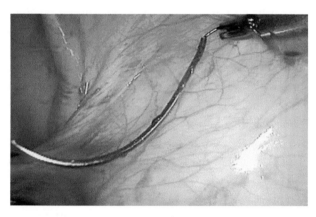

Figure 3.4 For needle removal, the suture is grasped within the needle-driver a few centimeters from the needle.

- For needle removal, the suture is grasped within the needle-driver a few centimeters from the needle; the suture is cut, and the needle is withdrawn into the introducer channel (Figure 3.4).

We use the standard two lateral trocars to perform laparoscopic suturing. The assistant holds the end of the suture and the surgeon forms the loop, or vice versa. It can be a simple knot or a surgical knot. Others perform knot-tying in a 'vertical zone' where they place two trocars on each side of the patient, with one surgeon performing the knot-tying.

EXTRACORPOREAL KNOT-TYING

For extracorporeal knot-tying, a knot-pusher (suture manipulator) is required, along with 70 cm suture length. It is easier to perform than intracorporeal knot-tying, but is not cost-effective. More importantly, the knot might not be as secure as with intracorporeal knot-tying, and the tissue could be pulled and traumatized.

- After placing the needle through the tissue, the suture is grasped a few centimeters from the needle and withdrawn from the abdominal cavity.
- The surgeon performs knot-tying extracorporeally. After each throw, the surgeon threads one end of the suture into the opening of the knot pusher (Figure 3.5). The other end of the suture remains free. The surgeon should apply equal tension to both ends of the suture, and the knot is slid down the trocar (Figures 3.6 and 3.7). This process is repeated to complete a surgical knot.

We do not recommend extracorporeal knot tying for tubal anastomosis, for other tuboplasty, or for suturing of the intestines (Figure 3.8). On the other hand, suturing of bleeding from a uterine perforation could be done using either intra- or extra-corporeal knot tying (Figure 3.9).

POTENTIAL COMPLICATIONS AND THEIR PREVENTION

- Injury to a vessel or bowel can occur. A mounted needle should be under vision all the time. It is better to remove a large needle (e.g., during a myomectomy) before knot-tying.
- The needle may be lost. Once the needle is separated from the suture, it has to be removed

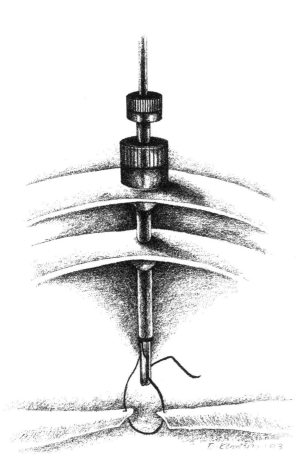

Figure 3.5 Extracorporeal knot-tying: withdrawal of the suture from the abdominal cavity by grasping it approximately 1 cm from the needle.

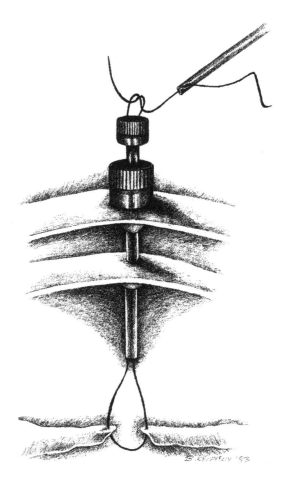

Figure 3.6 The needle is inserted into the fenestration of the knot-pusher before the knot is slid down into the abdominal cavity.

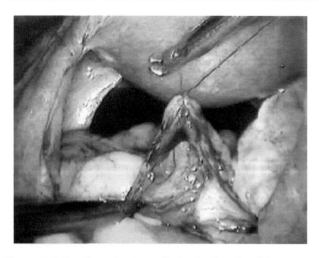

Figure 3.7 Equal tension is applied to both ends of the suture, and the knot is tightened with the help of the knot-pusher.

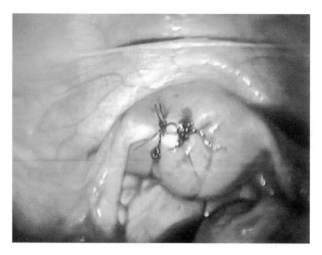

Figure 3.9 Bleeding uterine perforation has been closed with sutures.

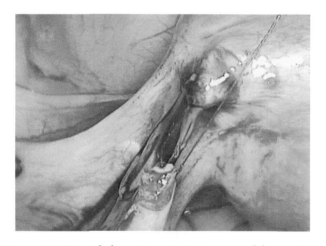

Figure 3.8 For tubal anastomosis, intracorporeal knot tying, should be used.

from the abdominal cavity. It is rare to lose a needle intraperitoneally. If the needle is not found, first examine the trocar sleeve. It is often located within the trap or impaled on a rubber washer. Otherwise, it might be caught on the peritoneum, including that of anterior abdominal wall.

SUGGESTED READING

- Koh C. Laparoscopic Suturing in the Vertical Zone. Tuttlingen: Endo-Press, 2004.

4

Laparoscopic tuboplasty with or without robotic assistance

Sejal Dharia Patel and Tommaso Falcone

Tubal disease represents one of the most important causes of infertility. Although most cases are secondary to sexually transmitted disease, tubal anastomosis represents a significant number of cases. Worldwide, more than 190 million couples have chosen sterilization as their contraceptive method. As many as 20% will express regret due to a change in family circumstances such as the death of a child, an improved economic situation, or a change in marital status; 1–5% of these patients will request sterilization reversal. Tubal disease amenable to surgical intervention can be divided into three approaches:

- cornual – which is treated radiologically or hysteroscopically and will not be covered in this chapter
- midportion – which is typically due to a previous tubal ligation
- distal tubal disease

For couples desiring fertility after tubal ligation, only two options are available: surgical tubal reanastomosis and in vitro fertilization. Tubal reanastomosis can be performed through a laparotomy incision, laparoscopically, or with robotic assistance. Integrated computer robotic systems allow for three-dimensional vision, tremor filtration, and intraabdominal articulation, affording the same advantages as laparo-tomy to the surgeon. Initial feasibility studies have been optimistic.

ROBOTIC TUBAL ANASTOMOSIS

Setup

1. The setup is similar to that for traditional laparoscopy.
2. The patient is placed in a modified dorsal lithotomy position in the Trendelenberg position.
3. The uterus is mobilized with an intrauterine cannula.
4. Peritoneal access is obtained using a 12 mm trocar through the umbilicus. Two lateral 8 mm ports (da Vinci ports, Intuitive Surgical, Inc.) are placed in the mid axillary line 2 cm below the umbilicus and separated by a minimum of 8 cm between port sites (Figure 4.1).
5. A fourth 10 mm accessory port can be placed on the left side between the umbilical and lateral ports to be used for irrigation, placement, and removal of sutures. A suprapubic port is sometimes used solely to introduce and remove needles.
6. A diagnostic laparoscopy is performed to assess the feasibility of the reanastomosis, with lysis of adhesions if necessary.
7. The robot is positioned between the patient's legs, and the robotic arms are connected to the respective ports.

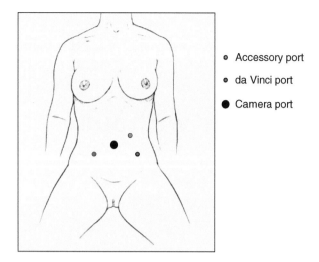

- ⊙ Accessory port
- ⊙ da Vinci port
- ● Camera port

Figure 4.1 Standard port placement for robotic tubal reanastomosis. The camera port (12 mm) is placed at the umbilicus. The da Vinci ports (8 mm) are placed in the midclavicular line, 1–2 cm below the level of the umbilicus, and lateral to the rectus muscle. Finally, an accessory port (10 mm) is positioned on the left side of patient, between the camera and the da Vinci port.

(a)

(b)

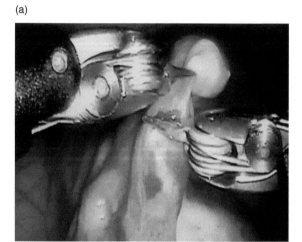

Figure 4.2 Preparation of the distal segment involves initially dissecting off the serosa 0.5 cm distally, and then creating a lumen. (Courtesy of Michael Steinkampf.)

PROCEDURE

1. Once the setup is completed, a robotic microforcep instrument and robotic microscissors are placed in both axillary ports.

2. Documentation of distal tubal patency before the anastomosis is important to prevent subsequent obstruction. This is done by using microforceps to compress the proximal portion of the distal segment to create a fluid pocket that can be incised and reveal the lumen. Alternatively, the proximal portion of the distal segment can be dilated with a 5 mm irrigation system to create a fluid pocket, which can be incised

3. The initial step is to prepare the distal tubal segment. This is done by stripping off its serosa using microscissors (Figure 4.2).

4. With the serosa stripped off, the tip is resected to express the lumen with protrusion of endosalpinx.

5. Attention is turned to the proximal segment. The microforceps can be switched for cautery, and the proximal segment is dissected free from the mesosalpinx (Figure 4.3).

6. The occluded segment is opened with laparoscopic endoshears placed in the axillary port.

7. Proximally, chromopertubation is used to demonstrate patency of the proximal tubal segment.

8. The mesosalpinx is approximated with interrupted 6-0 delayed absorbable (polyglactin) sutures, bringing the tubal segments in close proximity to prevent tension on the anastomosis.

9. The mucosa and muscular layers of the tubal segments are sutured with interrupted 7-0 Prolene (or polyglactin) sutures (Figure 4.4). The first suture is placed at 6 o'clock and tied.

10. The second suture is placed at 9 o'clock. This suture is not necessarily tied if the lumen is quite small.

11. The third and fourth sutures are placed at 12 o'clock and 3 o'clock, respectively. Then all sutures are tied. Either sutures can be placed

(a)

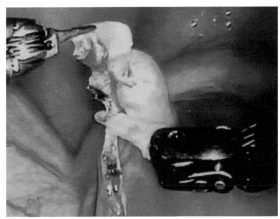

(b)

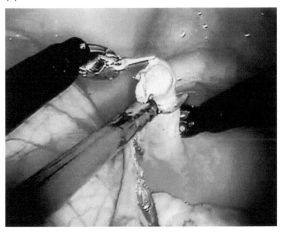

Figure 4.3 Preparation of the proximal segment involves initially incising and cauterizing the proximal mesosalpinx, and then transecting the proximal scarred segment to create a new lumen. (Courtesy of Michael Steinkampf.)

12. The serosa is closed separately with a running 7-0 Prolene suture (Figure 4.5).
13. Patency is determined by chromopertubation.
14. All ports ≥ 8 mm should be closed.

The final result of a robotically assisted tubal anastomosis is shown in Figure 4.6.

The procedure for tubal anastomosis without robotic assistance is illustrated in Figures 4.7–4.10.

FIMBRIOPLASTY

Procedure

1. The set-up and preliminary procedure are similar to those for tubal anastomosis.

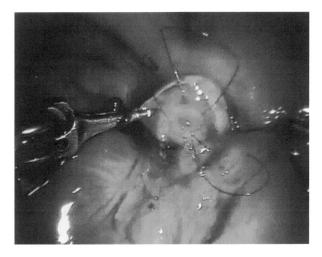

Figure 4.4 The inner layer includes a suture placed through the muscularis/mucosa in a running fashion at 12, 9, 6, and 3 o'clock. The sutures are then transected and ligated down individually. (Courtesy of Michael Steinkampf.)

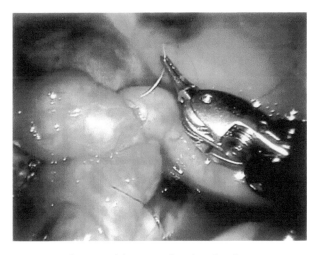

Figure 4.5 The serosal layer can be closed either in a running continuous fashion or using individual sutures. (Courtesy of Michael Steinkampf.)

2. The distal tube is grasped with an atraumatic forceps.
3. Lysis of the fimbrial adhesions is performed with fine scissors.
4. The laparoscope should be brought close to the fimbriae, and, with magnification, the fine adhesions that agglutinate the fimbriae are grasped and lysed.
5. If there is denser fimbrial phimosis, 6-0 polyglactin can be used to evert the edges.
6. If an antiadhesion barrier such as Interceed is used, care should be used not to enclose the tube and ovary together.

individually or one continuous suture can be used and the sutures cut after tying.

(a)

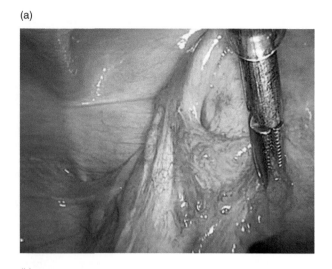

(b)

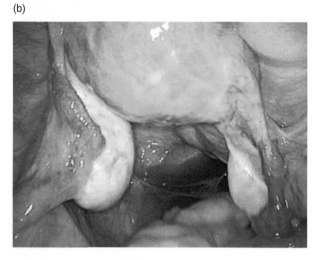

Figure 4.6 Fallopian tubes 1 year after robotically assisted anastomosis. (Courtesy of Michael Steinkampf.)

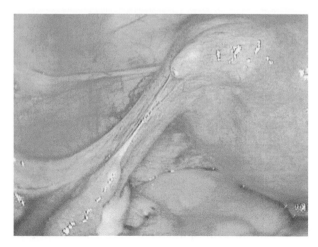

Figure 4.7 Tubal anastomosis without robotic assistance. (Courtesy of Togas Tulandi.)

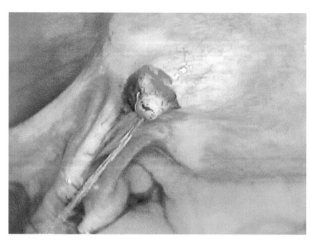

Figure 4.8

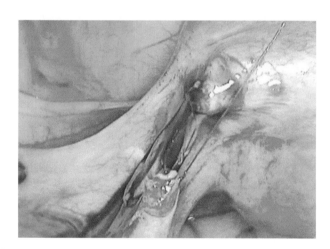

Figure 4.9

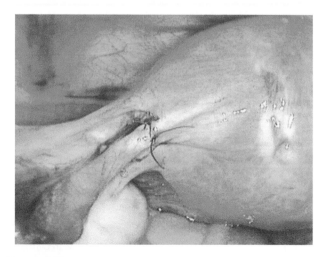

Figure 4.10

7. Fascia of the 5 mm ports do not have to be closed.

SALPINGOSTOMY

Procedure

1. The distal tube is grasped with an atraumatic forceps.
2. Lysis of the adhesions of the tube to the ovary, the pelvic sidewall, and sometimes the bowel should be performed with fine scissors.
3. Dilute indigo carmine dye is injected transcervically to distend the proximal tube. If there is a concomitant cornual block (bipolar occlusion), the procedure is terminated.
4. The distended distal segment is injected with dilute vasopressin (20 U/100 ml; this off-label use in the USA and the agent is not available in Europe).
5. The laparoscope should be brought close to the distended tube so that the surgery is performed under magnification.
6. An avascular scerotic line is usually identified, and is the incision point.
7. A scissors or microcautery set at 20 W pure-cut current can be used.
8. After making a cruciate-type incision, mucosal flaps are created.
9. Eversion of the mucosal flaps is performed using 6-0 Vicryl sutures. The suture is placed through the mucosa and out through the serosa. The suture is then placed into a nearby serosa and tied.
10. The presence or absence of mucosal folds, cilia, and fimbriae should be noted.

COMPLICATIONS AND THEIR PREVENTION

- Complications from robotically assisted surgery are similar to those of traditional laparoscopy with respect to injury to bowel, bladder, or major blood vessels.
- Specifically to robotically assisted surgery, injury can occur if the patient is not completely immobilized. The anesthesia team should be made aware of this risk, so that they can assure complete paralysis. In addition, the patient needs to be in optimal position (Trendelenberg, etc.) before docking of the robotic surgical system.
- During laparoscopic or robotic tubal reversals, removal of the fine needle and suture can be problematic. A laparoscopic needle-driver or a Maryland dissector can be used to remove the needle. The needle is usually grasped with the tip protected. In addition, the camera should follow the needle until it is in the port. Once the needle is removed from the abdomen, the bedside assistant should verbally confirm removal of the needle/suture. A magnetic blunt probe on the robotic instrument tray can be helpful to attract the needle to the anterior abdominal wall.
- Initially, operative times may exceed those for traditional open or laparoscopic approaches. This may result in periorbital edema or subcutaneous edema from prolonged Trendelenberg positioning.
- Bleeding from mesosalpingeal arteries in the mesosalpinx that lies inferior to the tubal lumen can pose a challenge in obtaining hemostasis. Micro-bipolar forceps will be beneficial to coagulate these vessels.

SUGGESTED READING

- Koh CH, Janik GM. Laparoscopic microsurgical tubal anastomosis. Obstet Gynecol Clin North Am 1999;26:189–200.
- Falcone T, Goldberg JM, Margossian H, Stevens L. Robotic-assisted laparoscopic microsurgical tubal anastomosis: a human pilot study. Fertil Steril 2000;73:1040–2.
- Degueldre M, Vandromme J, Huong PT, Cadiere GB. Robotically assisted laparoscopic microsurgical tubal reanastomosis: a feasibility study. Fertil Steril 2000;74:1020–3.
- Tulandi T, Collins JA, Burrows E. Treatment-dependent and treatment-independent pregnancy among women with periadnexal adhesions. Am J Obstet Gynecol 1990;162:354–7.

5

Ectopic pregnancy: Salpingostomy and salpingectomy

Pong Mo Yuen and Pui Shan Ng

The incidence of ectopic pregnancy has increased sixfold over the past 20 years in the developed countries. It is approximately 19 per 1000 pregnancies, with most cases occurring in the fallopian tube. This can be accounted for by the increase in the incidence of pelvic inflammatory disease and the use of assisted reproductive techniques. The incidence of ectopic pregnancy after in vitro fertilization can be as high as 4%.

Although there is an increasing trend toward treating tubal ectopic pregnancy with methotrexate, surgery is still needed in some cases, with laparoscopy being the preferred approach.

SALPINGOSTOMY

Due to the possibility of encountering hemoperitoneum, the surgeon should insert the laparoscope into the peritoneal cavity gradually (Figure 5.1). Otherwise, the lens will be stained with blood, which will impair visualization. Laparoscopic salpingostomy is most appropriate when the ectopic pregnancy implants in the ampullary portion of the tube (Figure 5.2). Isthmic ectopic pregnancy tends to grow through the lumen of the tube and erode the muscularis; tubal patency is therefore unlikely to be preserved, and there is a higher risk of persistent ectopic pregnancy.

Salpingostomy should be attempted if the patient wants to preserve fertility, especially when the contralateral tube is absent or diseased. The patient should be warned about the risks of persistent ectopic pregnancy and of recurrent ectopic pregnancy in

the future. Persistent ectopic pregnancy occurs in up to 5% of patients. Therefore, serum human chorionic genadotropin (hCG) level should be monitored following salpingostomy.

Procedure

1. Laparoscopy is performed in the usual fashion. The tube is immobilized with atraumatic grasping forceps. The mesosalpinx underneath the tubal pregnancy is infiltrated with either 5–10 ml of diluted epinephrine solution (1 in 200000) or vasopressin (1 IU diluted in 10 ml of normal saline) through a 22-gauge spinal needle or a laparoscopic injection needle (Figure 5.3). This will minimize bleeding and reduce the need for electrocoagulation.

2. A 1–2 cm linear incision is made at the area of maximal distention on the antemesosalpinx part of the tube (Figure 5.4). The incision can be performed using either a unipolar needle cautery at 30 W cutting current, a laser, or scissors. The products of conception are gently flushed out of the tube with a high pressure of irrigating solution (Figures 5.5 and 5.6). We do not recommend piecemeal removal of the products of conception with a grasping forceps, as this carries a high risk of persistent ectopic pregnancy. Care must be taken to avoid excessive evacuation, which will cause excessive bleeding and tubal damage. The tube is irrigated carefully and inspected for hemostasis.

3. The bleeding points can be controlled with micro-bipolar coagulation, but this should be as

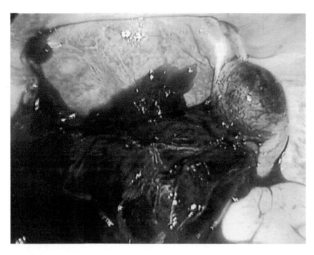

Figure 5.1 Due to the possibility of encountering hemoperitoneum, the laparoscope should be inserted into the peritoneal cavity gradually. (Courtesy of Togas Tulandi.)

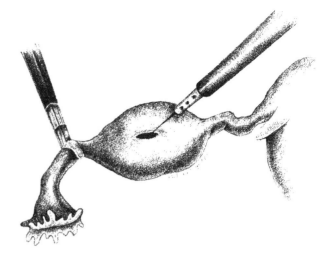

Figure 5.4 A longitudinal incision is made on the antemesosalpinx part of the tube.

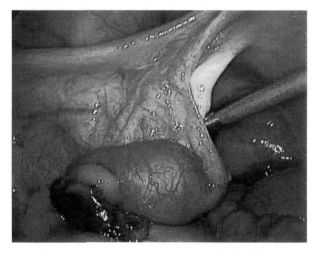

Figure 5.2 Ampullary pregnancy. (Courtesy of Togas Tulandi.)

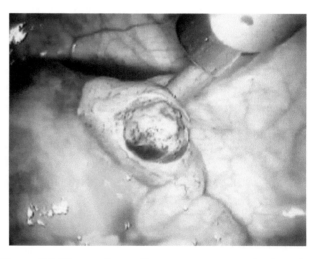

Figure 5.5 The products of conception are inside the tube. Note the blanching effects on the tissue of the vasopressin. (Courtesy of Togau Tulandi.)

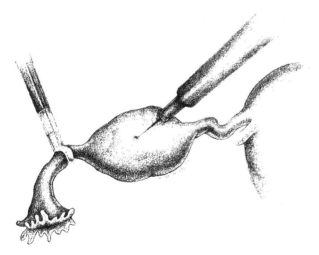

Figure 5.3 Linear salpingostomy: injection of vasopressin into the wall of the tube.

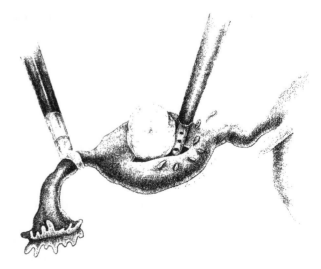

Figure 5.6 Flushing out the products of conception.

minimal as possible. Persistent bleeding from the placental bleeding can be controlled by injecting additional vasoconstricting solution and applying gentle pressure on the mesosalpinx. In the presence of persistent bleeding, two interrupted sutures of 4-0 PDS ligating the vessels in the mesosalpinx can be placed (Figure 5.7).

4. The tubal incision is left open to allow healing by secondary intention. The specimen is removed at the end of the operation through the trocar or by using an endoscopic pouch.

SALPINGECTOMY

Laparoscopic salpingectomy should be performed when future fertility is not desired, or in the case of a ruptured ectopic pregnancy with unstable hemodynamic status. Other indications include ectopic pregnancy following sterilization, a severely damaged tube, a large (≥ 4 cm) ectopic pregnancy, continuing hemorrhage following a salpingostomy, and chronic tubal pregnancy.

Procedure

1. In the presence of hemoperitoneum, the blood should be evacuated by suction irrigation. Blood clots are removed by applying continuous

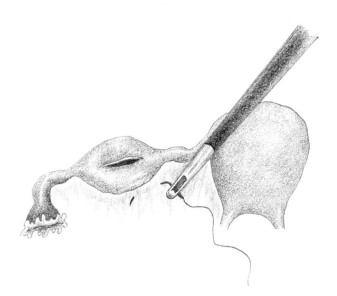

Figure 5.7 Suturing the vessels in the mesosalpinx using 4-0 polyglactin for persistent bleeding.

suction while moving the tip of the cannula in and out of the trocar sheath. The pelvic organs are irrigated with normal saline or lactated Ringer's solution.

2. The tube is grasped proximal or distal to the pregnancy and immobilized with atraumatic grasping forceps. Segmental resection of the tube or total salpingectomy can be performed, depending on the location of the pregnancy and the extent of tubal damage. Segmental resection is preferred when the pregnancy is in the isthmic part of the tube. It allows possible re-anastomosis later if desired. The tubal segment is excised by coagulating and cutting the tube proximal and distal to the pregnancy, followed by the mesosalpinx in between. One should avoid overcoagulating the tube, to minimize the thermal damage to the residual tube.

3. For total salpingectomy, the mesosalpinx from the fimbrial end is coagulated gradually and cut toward the isthmus. The excision should be performed close to the tube to avoid compromising the blood supply to the ovary. Care must be taken with the arcuate anastomosis branches of the ovarian and uterine vessels. The proximal tubal end should be completely desiccated with bipolar coagulation to eliminate the risk of fistula formation and subsequent tubal stump pregnancy. The procedure can also be performed using pretied suture or endoscopic loop (Endoloop) ligation of the tube, which is then transected above the ligation. It is generally recommended to apply two Endoloops to ensure complete hemostasis.

COMPLICATIONS AND THEIR PREVENTION

- Initial reports of laparoscopic salpingostomy revealed a rate of persistent ectopic pregnancy of 5–20%, which appears higher than the 2–11% after laparotomy. However, this could be related to the learning curve of the surgeons. It is more common when the pregnancy is in the proximal part of the fallopian tube and the products of conception are removed with forceps piecemeal. Weekly monitoring of serum hCG level after salpingostomy is needed to rule out persistent ectopic pregnancy. If the hCG level is rising or plateau, a methotrexate injection can be administered.

- Hemoperitoneum is not a contraindication for laparoscopy. Regardless of the surgical approach, an unstable patient must first be stabilized. An important consideration in deciding the surgical approach in women with bleeding ectopic pregnancy is the surgeon's expertise. Surgeons who perform advanced laparoscopic operations on a regular basis should be able to control the bleeding by laparoscopy in a short time. Otherwise, it will delay hemostasis.

SUGGESTED READING

- Tulandi T, Sammour A. Evidence-based management of ectopic pregnancy. Curr Opin Obstet Gynecol 2000;12:289–292.
- Sowter MC, Farquhar CM. Ectopic pregnancy: an update. Curr Opin Obstet Gynecol 2004;16:289–93.
- Royal College of Obstetricians and Gynaecologists. The Management of Tubal Pregnancy. Guideline No. 21. London: RCOG Press, 2004.
- Murray H, Baakdah H, Bardell T, Tulandi T. Diagnosis and treatmenst of ectopic pregnancy. CMAJ 2005;173:905–12.
- Hajenius PJ, Mol F, Mol BW, et al. Interventions for tubal ectopic pregnancy. Cochrane Database Syst Rev 2007;3(1):CD000324.

6

Ovarian cystectomy and oophorectomy

M Canis, R Botchorishvili, H Manhes, K Jardon, B. Rabischong, JL Pouly, and G Mage

The superiority of laparoscopic management of adnexal masses over laparotomy or even minilaparotomy has been shown in a few randomized trials. Due to the possibility of operating on undiagnosed ovarian cancer, and of spreading the tumor cells during surgery, special precautions should be taken. The initial and important step is to establish the diagnosis preoperatively. During surgery, benign tumors in young women should be treated conservatively, and malignant tumors should be staged immediately.

PROCEDURE

Diagnostic

Most ovarian cancers are diagnosed because of extraovarian signs of malignancy or obvious ultrasonographic appearance of malignancy. Otherwise, laparoscopy is a safe and reliable diagnostic tool. In the presence of a large pelvic mass, the secondary trocar should be inserted higher than the mass.

During surgery, the peritoneal fluid is aspirated for cytologic examination, and the entire peritoneal cavity is evaluated. One should not routinely puncture the cyst. However, if puncture is required, the internal cyst wall should then be examined for signs of malignancy. If the adnexa is removed intact, the surgeon and the pathologist should examine the inner cyst wall immediately after removal.

Laparoscopic puncture

Care should be taken to minimize spillage when puncturing a cyst. First, the adnexa is stabilized by placing an atraumatic forceps on the utero-ovarian ligament. The puncture is performed on the anti-mesenteric border of the ovary, perpendicular to the ovarian surface (Figure 6.1). Small cysts are aspirated with a needle connected to a 20 ml syringe (Figures 6.1 and 6.2). Larger cysts of (>5 cm) are punctured with a 5 mm conical trocar and emptied with a suction–irrigator (Figures 6.3 and 6.4). A 5 mm trocar is used because, or comparison with to the use of cutting instruments, the puncture is almost water-tight, and drainage is faster.

Because minimal spillage still occurs, a large endo-pouch should be placed in the pelvis, and the ovary punctured inside the pouch. This technique is not feasible for large adnexal masses > 8 cm or in patients with severe pelvic adhesions (Figure 6.4).

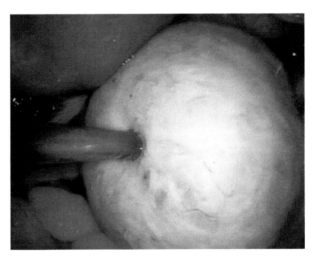

Figure 6.1 Puncture of a benign cyst on the antimesenteric border using a laparoscopic needle.

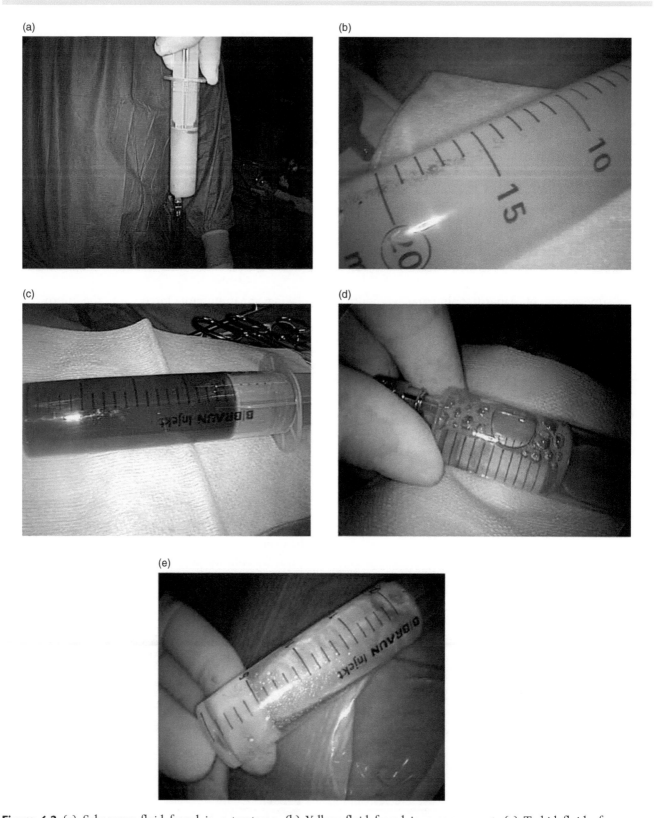

Figure 6.2 (a) Sebaceous fluid found in a teratoma. (b) Yellow fluid found in a serous cyst. (c) Turbid fluid of a serous low-malignant-potential tumor. (d) Safran yellow fluid of a functional cyst. (e) Clear fluid of a paraovarian cyst or a benign serous ovarian cyst.

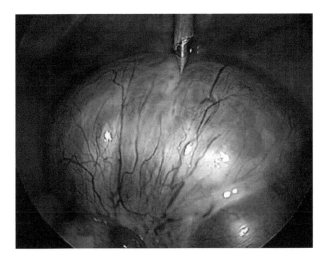

Figure 6.3 Puncture with a 5 mm conical trocar.

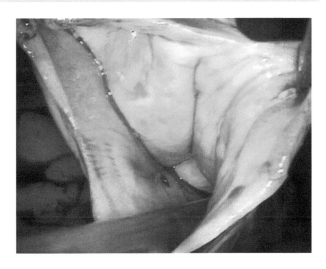

Figure 6.5 Intracystic inspection.

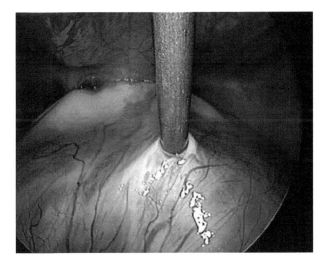

Figure 6.4 Aspiration of the cyst content using a 5 mm aspiration lavage device.

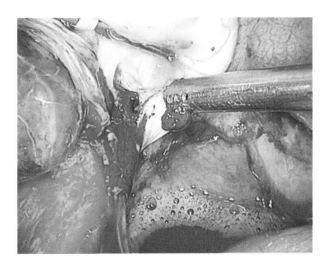

Figure 6.6 Adhesiolysis of a left ovarian endometrioma.

Inspection of cyst fluid and intracystic examination

The cyst fluid is sent for cytologic examination (Figure 6.2). Lavage of the cyst and the pelvic cavity is performed several times with a small volume of fluid to avoid contamination of the upper abdomen. The cyst is opened with scissors and the internal cyst wall carefully inspected (Figure 6.5). If suspicious findings are present, the cyst is treated as malignant.

Ovarian cystectomy

- Following decompression of an ovarian cyst, the cyst wall and the ovarian tissue retract to different degrees, and a cleavage plane develops spontaneously (Figure 6.7).

- The cyst wall is separated from the ovarian tissue using grasping forceps with teeth (Figure 6.8). We use two grasping forceps side by side: one holds the cyst wall and another the ovarian tissue. The forceps are pulled in opposite directions until the cyst wall is detached from the ovarian tissue.

- Hemostasis should be performed during dissection. It is more difficult to secure the bleeding at the completion of dissection, when the ovarian tissue has retracted.

- To avoid ovarian damage, one should follow the proper cleavage plane. This plane is reached when the outer surface of the cyst wall appears white. Red fibrotic tissue on the cyst wall indicates an incorrect plane (Figure 6.9).

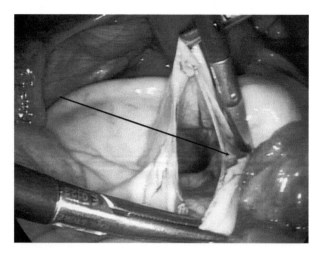

Figure 6.7 After incision of the ovary, the cleavage plane is easily identified (arrow).

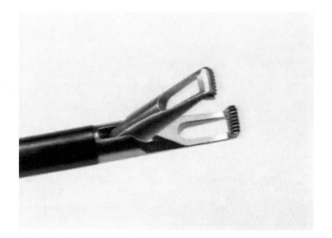

Figure 6.8 Atraumatic grasping forceps.

Paraovarian cysts

These have transparent thin walls and appear bluish (Figure 6.10). If vegetations are present, the cyst wall looks thick and white. In this case, the cyst should not be punctured (Figure 6.10).

Endometriomas

These can be treated by fenestration and ablation with a carbondioxide laser or bipolar coagulation, or by cystectomy. Cystectomy is associated with a lower recurrence rate and higher pregnancy rate in infertile women. We propose the following surgical steps:

1. Obtaining fluid for cytology and a thorough examination of the peritoneal cavity.

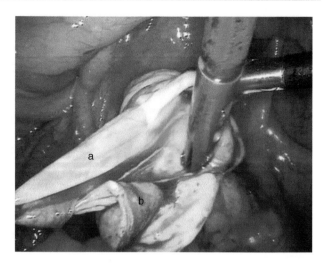

Figure 6.9 (a) In this part of the dissection, the cyst wall is white – the plane is correct. (b) In this part, red fibers are visible on the surface of the cyst – a better plane was found (see zone a).

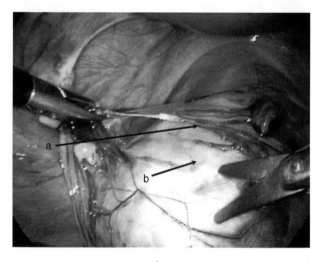

Figure 6.10 Dissection of a paraovarian cyst: the peritoneum (a) is opened before dissection of the plane (b).

2. Liberation of the ovary from the broad ligament. In most cases, endometriomas are fixed to the broad ligament. As the adhesions involve the endometrioma itself, the cyst often ruptures during liberation (Figure 6.6). If puncturing of the cyst is needed, it should be performed on the anterior surface, and after adhesiolysis.

3. Lavage of the cyst wall and the pelvic cavity.

4. Endocystic examination.

5. Identification of the cleavage plane by enlarging the ovarian incision.

6. Separation of the cyst wall from the ovarian tissue.

7. Dissection using the stripping technique in the incorrect plane would remove the fibrosis, induce bleeding, and damage the ovary. To avoid this scenario, it is necessary or find the proper cleavage plane close to the cyst wall. Two grasping forceps are used to expose the plane. Bipolar coagulation and scissors are used to cut the red fibrotic fibers on the surface of the cyst, facilitating identification of the cleavage plane. The plane is found by following the red 'arrows' of fibrotic tissue (Figures 6.11 and 6.12).

8. Hemostasis is achieved with bipolar coagulation, and the final shape of the ovary is checked. One intraovarian suture is used if the ovary is gaping.

9. The cyst wall is extracted using an Endobag (Karl Storz, Tutlingen, Germany).

Dermoid cysts

The ovary is grasped on its antimesenteric surface with atraumatic forceps. A small superficial incision of the ovarian cortex is performed with scissors. Then aquadissection may be used through this small incision, and the incision is enlarged carefully. The plane is developed with atraumatic grasping forceps or with scissors (Figures 6.13 and 6.14). Most cases of rupture occur while enlarging the incision, even though the cleavage plane has been identified. This occurs especially with cysts >8 cm.

To avoid rupture, the dissection should be performed without grasping the cyst or pushing it, and with the instruments being used parallel to the ovarian surface. Alternatively, one can place the cyst in an Endobag (Ethicon Endo-Surgery, Inc.) before dissection.

Laparoscopic adnexectomy (Figures 6.15 and 6.16)

To remove the ovary, surgeons have a choice between oophorectomy and adnexectomy. As it is important to

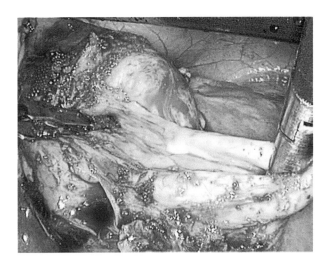

Figure 6.12 When the fibrotic 'arrow' is cut, the correct plane is found.

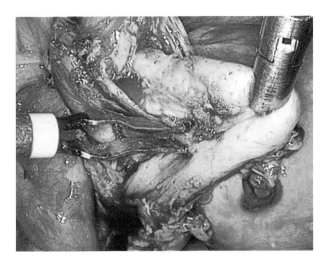

Figure 6.11 A red 'arrow' of fibrotic tissue is showing where the plane should be looked for. The top of this 'arrow' is coagulated.

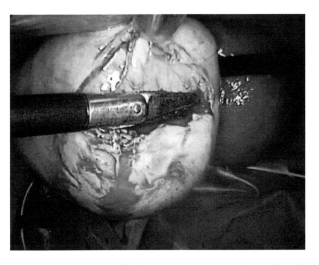

Figure 6.13 Incision of the ovarian cortex: the yellow fat content of the teratoma is clearly seen; the scissors are parallel to the surface of the cyst.

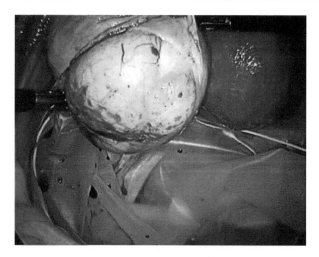

Figure 6.14 Cystectomy without puncture for a benign teratoma: the forceps are moved away from the cyst surface.

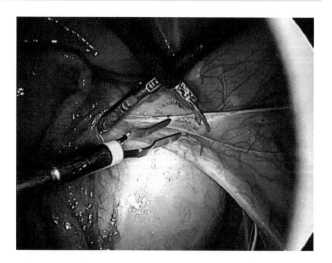

Figure 6.15 The infundubulopelvic ligament is pulled medially with atraumatic forceps, and the peritoneum is opened lateral to the ovarian vessels.

remove the entire ovary, and hemostasis of the ovarian hilum is more difficult than that of the adnexal vessels, in our institution we do not perform oophorectomy alone.

- The procedure is usually simple; however, it becomes difficult when the ovary is adherent to the broad ligament with dense adhesions. In such cases, an removal of the posterior leaf of the broad ligament is required to ensure complete removal of the ovarian tissue and to avoid the risks of ovarian remnant syndromes. To achieve this, the ureter is identified on the pelvic brim and dissected down to the uterine vessels (Figures 6.17 and 6.18). When the ovary is stuck to the broad ligament, complete dissection of the ureter is required. This dissection is particularly important and difficult in patients with endometriosis, since it frequently invades the retroperitoneal space, and the ureter may be involved in the fibrosis (Figure 6.18).

- Hemostasis of the adnexal vessels can be achieved either with bipolar coagulation or with sutures (Figures 6.16 and 6.19). We use bipolar coagulation in most cases. Stapling devices present no advantages. Opening the peritoneum between the ovarian vessels and the round ligament facilitates ligation of the vessels in the infundibulopelvic ligament (Figure 6.15). The posterior leaf of the broad ligament can be opened as well if needed. Accordingly, the ovarian vessels

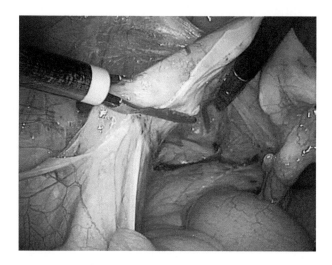

Figure 6.16 Left adnexectomy: bipolar coagulation is applied on the vessels after dissection of the peritoneum.

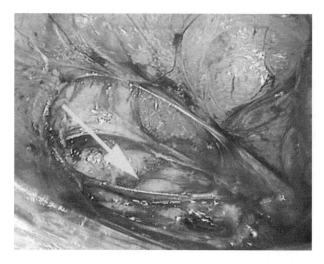

Figure 6.17 The left ureter is visible after dissection of the retroperitoneal area.

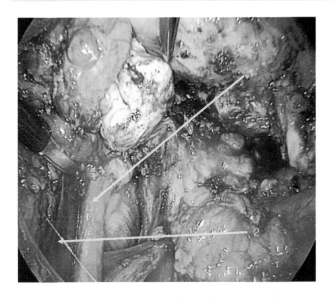

Figure 6.18 Left adnexectomy for endometriosis: the ureter (1) has been dissected to excise the peritoneum of the broad ligament (2).

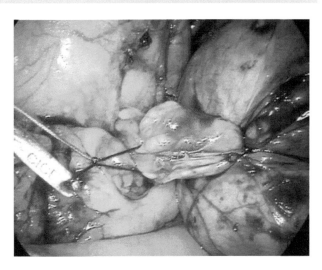

Figure 6.19 Hemostasis of ovarian vessels using a knot-pusher.

can be stretched more than when they are covered by the peritoneum. In addition, direct coagulation on the vessels is more effective (Figure 6.16).

Specimen removal

- Due to the possibility of contamination of abdominal wall with cancer cells or endometriosis, the use of an endoscopic pouch is mandatory. The ideal endoscopic pouch should be large enough for specimen removal without enlarging the incision, should be easy to open, and should remain open in the abdominal cavity for a sufficiently long time to allow easy extraction in obese patients. It should also be strong, and transparent to allow visual control of puncture procedures performed in the pouch.
- We use an Endobag (Figure 6.20). The bag is extracted either through a 10 mm port on the right low abdominal quadrant or through the umbilical incision (Figures 6.21 and 6.22). An Endobag is required even if the mass is extracted through the vagina.
- Large cysts require puncturing or draining before extraction. We puncture the cyst through the abdominal wall after extraction of the neck of the

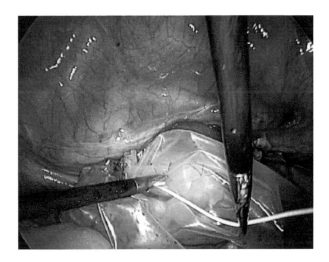

Figure 6.20 Closing an Endobag.

bag (Figure 6.23). It is important to puncture inside the bag – not through it.

- Alternatively, the specimen can be extracted through a colpotomy incision on the posterior cul-de-sac. We use an instrument designed by the Lausanne group, which allows the posterior fornix to be opened and the bag grasped without losing the pneumoperitoneum (Figures 6.24 and 6.25).
- When an adnexectomy is performed concomitant with a hysterectomy, the adnexectomy is performed first. The mass is placed in a closed bag in the paracolic gutter for extraction after the hysterectomy.

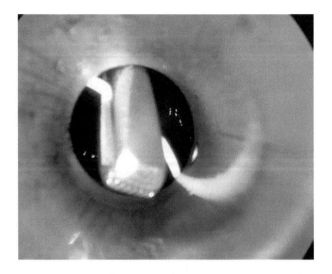

Figure 6.21 The Endobag is pushed through the umbilical trocar.

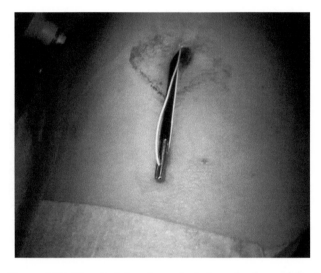

Figure 6.22 The Endobag is pushed through the umbilical incision; the umbilical trocar has been removed.

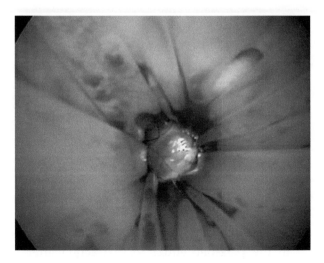

Figure 6.23 Puncture of the cyst in the Endobag.

Suturing

A small ovarian opening can be approximated by light application of bipolar coagulation or the ovarian cortex (Figure 6.26). Large defects need to be sutured with one or two intraovarian sutures.

COMPLICATIONS AND THEIR PREVENTION

- Spillage of cystic contents should be minimized by using an endoscopic pouch. Besides the possibility of dissemination of cancer cells, spillage

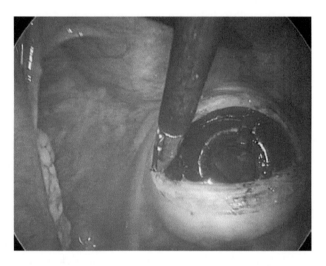

Figure 6.24 Laparoscopic colpotomy using the Spuhler instrument.

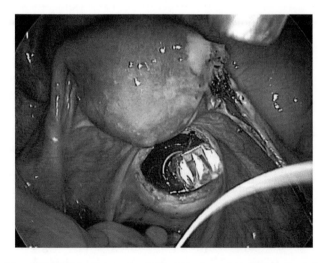

Figure 6.25 The bag is grasped with a forceps inserted through the vagina, using the same instrument.

(a)

(b)

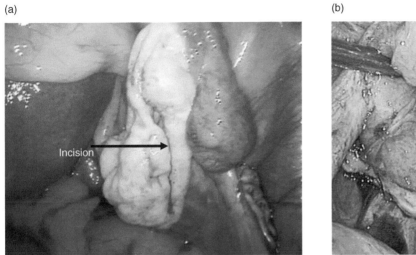

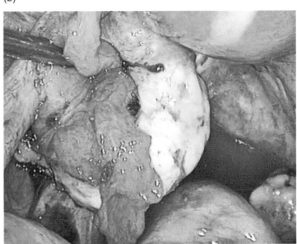

Figure 6.26 Final view after dissection of a serous cyst (a) and of an endometrioma (b).

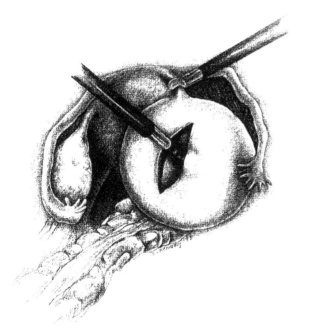

Figure 6.27 Creating a cleavage plane by injecting physiologic saline into the ovarian capsule.

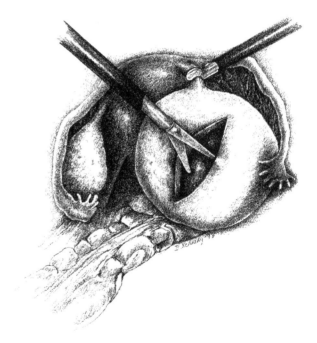

Figure 6.28 A superficial incision is made on the ovarian capsule without entering the cyst.

of dermoid cystic contents is associated with peritoneal granulomatosis in 1% of cases. Endometriosis on the abdominal wall following extraction without a pouch has also been reported.

• A gaping ovary predisposes to adhesion formation, including trapping a loop of bowel inside. Suturing of the ovarian opening is recommended.

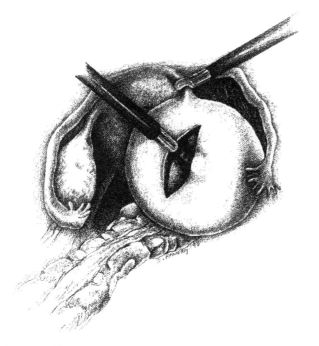

Figure 6.29

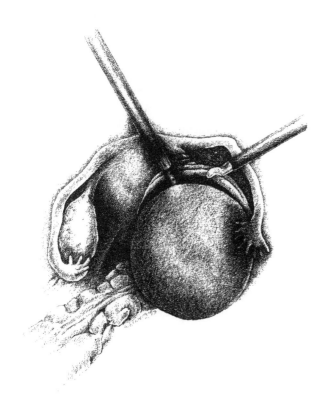

Figure 6.30

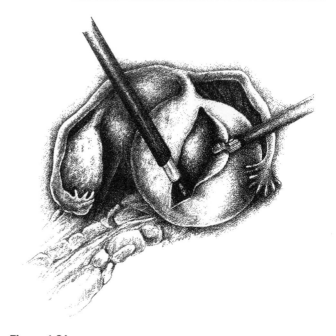

Figure 6.31

Figure 6.29, 6.30, 6.31 Enucleation of the cyst using hydrodissection.

SUGGESTED READING

- Panici PB, Muzii L, Palaia I, et. al. Minilaparotomy versus laparoscopy in the treatment of benign adnexal cysts: a randomized clinical study. Eur J Obstet Gynecol Reprod Biol 2007; in press.
- Jones KD, Fan A, Sutton CJ. The ovarian endometrioma: Why is it so poorly managed? Indicators from an anonymous survey. Hum Reprod 2002;17:845–9.
- Canis M, Mage G, Wattiez A, Pouly JL, Bruhat MA. The ovarian endometrioma: Why is it so poorly managed? Laparoscopic treatment of large ovarian endometrioma: Why such a long learning curve? Hum Reprod 2003;18:5–7.
- Canis M, Rabischong B, Houlle C, et. al. Laparoscopic management of adnexal masses: a gold standard? Curr Opin Obstet Gynecol 2002;14:423–8.
- Canis M, Mashiach R, Wattiez A, et. al. Frozen section in laparoscopic management of macroscopically suspicious ovarian masses. J Am Assoc Gynecol Laparosc 2004;11:365–9.
- Hart RJ, Hickey M, Maouris P, Buckett W, Garry R. Excisional surgery versus ablative surgery for ovarian endometriomata. Cochrane Database Syst Rev 2005;(3):CD004992.

7

Laparoscopic treatment of ovarian remnant

Camran Nezhat, Ceana Nezhat, and Farr Nezhat

Ovarian remnants occur when ovarian tissue is inadvertently left in the pelvic cavity after oophorectomy. The remaining functional ovarian tissue can respond to hormonal stimulation with growth, cystic degeneration, or hemorrhage, and produces pain. Predisposing factors include increased vascularity causing difficult hemostasis, endometriosis, pelvic inflammatory disease, pelvic adhesions, multiple previous operations, and altered anatomy. Other factors associated with ovarian remnants are the use of endoscopic loops for laparoscopic oophorectomy, multiple operative procedures with incomplete removal of pelvic organs, densely adherent ovaries, and multiple ovarian cystectomies for functional cysts. When pretied sutures or stapling devices are used for the infundibulopelvic ligament, they should be placed well below the ovarian tissue.

Ovarian remnants are usually encased in adhesions (Figure 7.1). It is not unusual for these patients to have undergone previous attempts to excise the tissue. Symptoms of ovarian remnant usually occur within 5 years of oophorectomy. The most frequent symptom is pelvic pain. This varies from cyclic to chronic pain, dull and aching to sharp and stabbing. Imaging studies, including vaginal ultrasound, computed tomography (CT), and magnetic resonance imaging (MRI), are useful but not always indicative of ovarian remnant. Preoperative follicle-stimulating hormone (FSH) levels can contribute to the diagnosis when found in the premenopausal range ($<$40 IU/l) in patients who have undergone bilateral oophorectomy. Ovarian stimulation can be used to increase the volume of the ovarian remnant, helping to confirm the

diagnosis preoperatively or facilitating the search of the tissue intraoperatively. Laparoscopic ultrasonography can be helpful in detecting ovarian remnants in patients with distorted pelvic anatomy.

PROCEDURE

Surgical excision of the ovarian remnant by laparoscopy is the best choice in most cases. It is imperative that the patient undergo a thorough 1- or 2-day bowel prep (both mechanical and antibiotic). The patient should be carefully consented regarding the possibility of proctosigmoidoscopy, cystoscopy, or resection of a portion of the bowel, bladder, or ureters, as well as the possibility of conversion to laparotomy. With ovarian

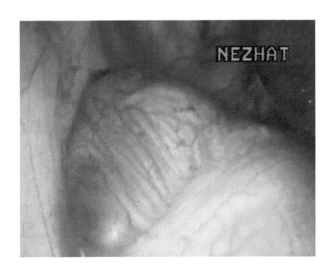

Figure 7.1 Ovarian remnant encased in adhesions.

remnant, the patient must understand that the goal is complete resection of the ovarian tissue in order to prevent recurrences.

Due to the possibility of encountering anterior abdominal wall adhesions, we recommend an open laparoscopy, right upper quadrant entry, or mapping technique. After insertion of all the instruments, intraabdominal adhesions are lysed and normal anatomy is restored as much as possible. The ovarian remnant is identified and dissected. Extensive and careful retroperitoneal dissection is required to facilitate identification and removal of the ovarian tissue.

Ovarian remnant adherent to lateral pelvic wall

When the ovarian remnant is adherent to the lateral pelvic wall (Figure 7.2), we use hydrodissection with lactated Ringer's solution to create a cleavage plane. The peritoneum is opened to the infundibulopelvic ligament of the ovarian remnant. Even in cases with retroperitoneal fibrosis, the combination of hydrodissection and sharp dissection with a carbon dioxide (CO_2) laser is usually successful. Adhesions are lysed until the course of the major pelvic blood vessels and the ureter can be traced and, if necessary, dissected. The ovarian blood supply is coagulated with bipolar forceps, and the ovarian tissue is excised and submitted for histologic examination. When the ovarian remnant is adhered to the vaginal cuff and the bladder (Figure 7.3), deep dissection and extensive ureterolysis are not necessary; however, identification of the anatomy and a plane of dissection is essential.

Ovarian remnant adherent to the bowel

When the remnant is adherent to the bowel (Figure 7.4), adhesions are lysed using hydrodissection and the CO_2 laser or sharp dissection with harmonic devices or similar modalities. Ovarian tissue embedded in the superficial muscularis of the bowel is removed with a shaving technique. When the remnant is deeply embedded in the bowel or bladder muscularis or when the ureter is involved or possibly obstructed, partial removal of the structure and repair are necessary. The serosa and muscularis layers are reinforced with one to three interrupted 4-0 polydioxanone or polyglactin sutures in one layer. Sigmoidoscopy and examination underwater are used to confirm that the repair is airtight. Bipolar forceps or sealing devices are used to desiccate the ovarian blood supply and the

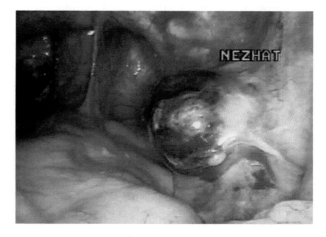

Figure 7.2b

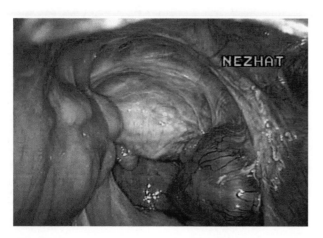

Figure 7.2a Ovarian remnant adherent to the lateral pelvic wall.

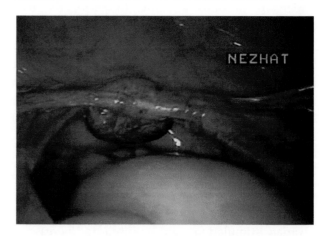

Figure 7.3a Ovarian remnant adhered to the vaginal Cuff.

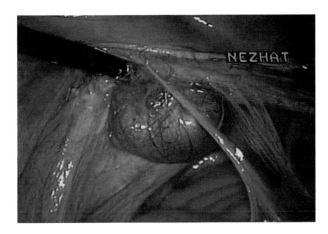

Figure 7.3b

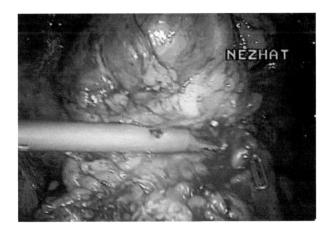

Figure 7.4 Ovarian remnant adhered to the bowel.

ovarian remnant, and the contiguous peritoneum and surrounding tissue are meticulously excised and submitted for histologic examination.

A variety of findings, including follicular cysts, endometriosis, corpus luteum, and ovarian cancer, have been found in the ovarian remnant tissue. In fact, there are five documented cases of ovarian cancer developing in an ovarian remnant after total abdominal hysterectomy and bilateral salpingo-oophorectomy.

COMPLICATIONS AND THEIR PREVENTION

The incidence of injury to the bladder, ureter, and bowel at laparotomy for ovarian remnant is estimated to be 3–33%, with injuries to the ureter being significantly greater with laparotomy than with laparoscopy. The following are key steps to safe, complete resection of ovarian remnant:

1. The anatomy should be restored as completely as possible with bilateral sidewall and cul-de-sac dissection. Any other pelvic pathology, such as endometriosis, should be treated.
2. The ureter should be identified and dissected completely – to the pelvic brim, if necessary. The value of ureteral stenting is controversial.
3. There must be complete excision of the ovarian remnant, including a wide margin of healthy tissue. Resection of the adherent structures, such as portions of bowel or bladder, may be necessary to resect the tissue completely – this is to prevent recurrence.
4. The ovary should be removed in one piece, placed in a surgical specimen bag, and extracted from the abdominal cavity through an enlarged trocar site, posterior colpotomy, or large cannula. However, in patients with severe endometriosis and paraovarian adhesions, the ovary may be fragmented and removed in pieces, and great care must be taken to ensure complete removal. Note that the devascularized ovarian tissue can reimplant on peritoneal surfaces.
5. Complete and thorough examination of the abdominal cavity should be performed before completing the procedure, to identify any other possible sites of ovarian remnant.

SUGGESTED READING

- Orford V, Kuhn R. Management of ovarian remnant syndrome. Aust NZ J Obstet Gynaecol 1996; 36:468–71.
- Minke T, DePond W, Winkelmann T, Blythe J. Ovarian remnant syndrome: study in laboratory rats. Am J Obstet Gynecol 1994;171:1440.

- Nezhat CH, Kearney S, Malik S, Nezhat C, Nezhat F. Laparoscopic management of ovarian remnant. Fertil Steril 2005;83:973–8.
- Nezhat F, Nezhat C, Nezhat CH, et al. Use of laparoscopic ultrasonography to detect ovarian remnants. Am J Obstet Gynecol 1996;174:641.
- Narayansingh G, Cumming G, Parkin D, Miller I. Ovarian cancer developing in the ovarian remnant syndrome. A case report and literature review. Aust NZ J Obstet Gynaecol 2000;40:221–3.

8

Laparoscopic excision of endometriosis

Philippe R Koninckx

The best treatment of endometriosis remains surgery. However, the surgery and definition of endometriosis have changed over time (Figure 8.1). For example, surgeons are more aware of the subtle appearance of endometriosis (Figures 8.2 and 8.3), as well as 'unrecognized' deep endometriosis (Figure 8.4). Reporting the depth and volume of deep endometriosis is necessary to evaluate results of surgery. Similarly, the size of ovarian endometriomas, the presence of adhesions, the pathologic confirmation of the disease, and the technique used, are essential to compare results of different type operations for endometriosis.

We believe that the carbon dioxide (CO_2) laser is a precise cutting instrument with minimal resultant tissue damage. On the other hand, electrosurgery is more versatile in coagulation and cutting, but it is slower. Another difference between laser and electrosurgery is the angle of energy delivery to the tissue. A laser beam through the laparoscope has an almost horizontal delivery to the rectovaginal septum, whereas electrical energy though the secondary trocar has a more vertical line of delivery. Two secondary trocars would be sufficient for simple laser surgery for endometriosis, and they are placed low in the abdomen. For electrosurgery, we use three secondary trocars, which, ergonomically, have to be placed high on43 the abdomen.

MINIMAL AND MILD ENDOMETRIOSIS

Procedure

We vaporize endometriosis lesions with high power of the CO_2 laser, and excise large lesions. If a CO_2 laser is unavailable, one can use electrosurgery. Sharp excision with electrosurgery balances between extensive coagulation for hemostasis and minimal coagulation, which could be associated with capillary bleeding and poor visualization. Bipolar coagulation should not be used for vaporization, since the depth of infiltration and of coagulation are both difficult to evaluate.

CYSTIC OVARIAN ENDOMETRIOSIS

Procedure

The results of laparoscopy and of laparotomy– microsurgical treatment of cystic ovarian endometriosis are comparable (Figure 8.5). The rate of pain relief is 60–80% and the cumulative pregnancy rate is 60–70% at 6 to12 months after surgery. The recurrence rate of cystic lesions is 5–7% after excision, but is much higher (20%) after local aspiration. Ultrasound-guided aspiration results in massive intraabdominal spillage of the 'chocolate material.' We do not recommend these techniques.

- In our institution, we strip or excise the cyst wall (Figures 8.6 and 8.7). This is a fast and complete treatment. Following adhesiolysis, drainage, and rinsing of the cyst content, we incise the ovarian capsule around the cyst opening with the CO_2 laser. Once a cleavage plane is found, we strip the cyst wall from the ovary. We use the laser to prevent tearing the ovarian capsule and to assist stripping, especially at the level of the ovarian hilum.

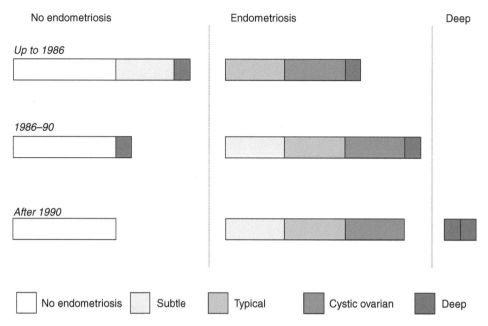

Figure 8.1 What is understood by the word 'endometriosis' has varied over time.

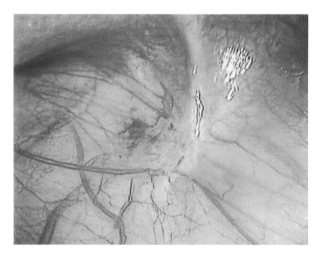

Figure 8.2 Subtle appearance of endometriosis. (Courtesy of Togas Tulandi.)

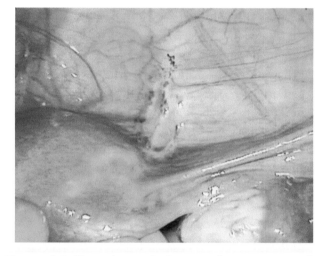

Figure 8.3 Classical powder-burn endometriosis in the anterior cul-de-sac. (Courtesy of Togas Tulandi.)

- Some authors have reported closure of the ovary with surgical glue or sutures when the remaining ovarian flaps are unequal in size. Laser vaporization or electrocoagulation of the inner cyst wall has been shown to be effective; however, it was not possible to judge the thermal injury. Superficial destruction results in high recurrence rates, whereas deep destruction often causes bleeding.
- For large cyst >5 cm, the size and the thin ovarian capsule precludes excision and/or vaporization. Therefore, either an adnexectomy or a two-step surgery should be performed.
  - The first step is to create a large window in the cyst wall, rinsing and draining the content of the cyst, followed by a 3-month treatment with gonadotropin-releasing hormone (GnRH) agonists.
  - We perform the second step of the procedure if the cyst persists. They consists of excision of the cyst – which has become smaller, thus facilitating the procedure.

(a)

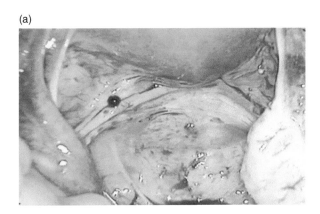

(b)

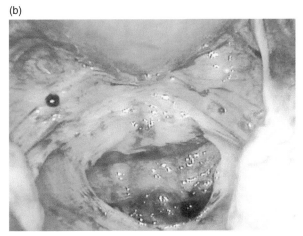

Figure 8.4 Deep infiltrating endometriosis in the posterior cul-de-sac before (a) and after (b) excision. (Courtesy of Togas Tulandi.)

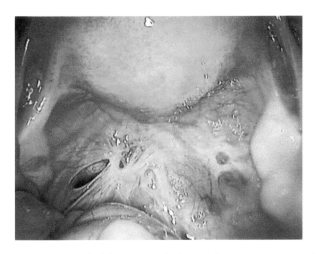

Figure 8.5 Partial obliteration of the cul-de-sac. (Courtesy of Togas Tulandi.)

Complications and their prevention

- Preserving an intact ovary requires careful dissection in order not to tear off part of the capsule or the red fibers attached to the cyst.

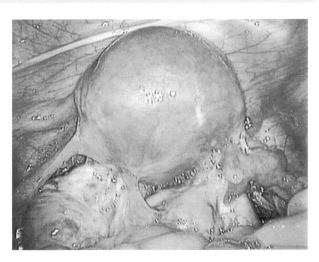

Figure 8.6 Bilateral ovarian endometriomas (Kissing ovaries) with adhesions. (Courtesy of Togas Tulandi.)

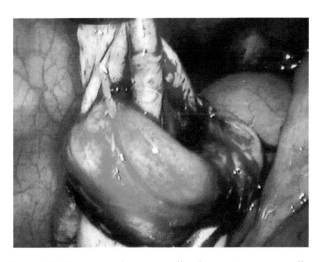

Figure 8.7 Stripping the cyst wall. The ovarian cyst wall is under traction; the pink area is the inner side of the ovary. (Courtesy of Togas Tulandi.)

- To prevent injury to the blood vessels in the hilum, the surgeon should perform meticulous dissection. Otherwise extensive coagulation is needed devascularizing the ovary. We consider this a technically difficult and delicate surgery – more so than advanced lymph node dissection.

DEEP ENDOMETRIOSIS

Definitions

We believe that 'adenomyotic nodule' is a better terminology for deep endometriosis. The lesion is generally large, homogeneous on histopathology, and clonal in origin (like cystic ovarian endometriosis).

It can infiltrate the surrounding tissue, resulting in sclerotic and inflammatory reaction with bowel stenosis or ureteral obstruction. The most severe forms are rectovaginal endometriosis and endometriosis invading the sigmoid colon.

The surgeon should make a diagnosis before surgery. If a rectovaginal nodule is suspected, we perform a contrast enema and an intravenous pyelography (IVP). If the IVP reveals a hydronephrosis, preoperative stents are placed. If the diameter of the sigmoid is reduced by <50% over a length <2.5 cm, we plan a discoid excision and for larger sigmoid lesions, a resection and anastomosis. For rectal involvement, we plan a discoid excision as well. Magnetic resonance imaging (MRI) and computed tomography (CT) scan add little to the clinical management. Preoperatively, a bowel preparation is given.

Procedure (Figures 8.8–8.15)

1. First, the ovaries are liberated from the ovarian fossa. In difficult cases, the ovaries can be sutured to the abdominal wall, facilitating visualization.
2. The sigmoid colon is separated from the sidewall. In the presence of an adenomyotic nodule, it is cut in half without attempting to dissect it from the sidewall or from the sigmoid. The surgeon should take time to mobilize the rectum and sigmoid out of the pelvis. These organs are then sutured to the peritoneum with one or two sutures, as for promontofixation. This approach enhances exposure without the need for an extreme Trendelenburg position, and it frees one of the assistant's hands.
3. We believe that the CO_2 laser facilitates surgery in the presence of frozen pelvis and bilateral endometriomas.
4. The course of the ureter should be followed. If necessary, ureterolysis is performed, with excision of endometriosis and dissection of the adenomyotic nodule. Here, the dissection is done with scissors and electrosurgery.
5. Excision of the rectovaginal nodule is performed by following the lateral and posterior margins of the nodule up to the pararectal space. Dissection of large nodules around the ischial spine and deep lateral dissection up to the vaginal wall have

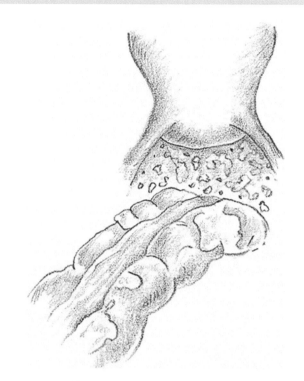

Figure 8.8 Diffuse endometriosis of the posterior culde-sac.

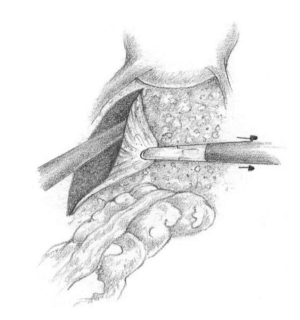

Figure 8.9 A peritoneal incision has been made just medial to the left uterosacral ligament, and blunt dissection underneath and traction on the peritoneum allows the resection to begin.

to be done thoroughly. This is to minimize bleeding and to preserve the parasympathetic nerve.
6. The endometriotic nodule is separated from the rectum down to the muscularis. When it is deeper than the muscularis, excision is performed with

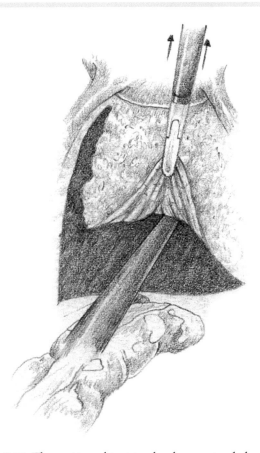

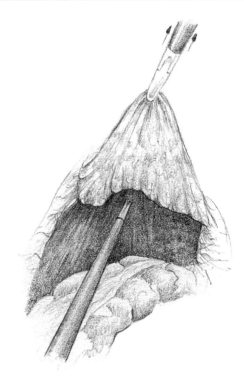

Figure 8.11 Blunt dissection is used to continue to lift the peritoneum off of the rectum. When tendrils of connective tissue are visible, they can be safely severed with laser or electrosurgery.

Figure 8.10 The peritoneal incision has been extended across the cul-de-sac adjacent to the rectum, and traction and blunt dissection allow the peritoneum to be lifted off the underlying rectum. The longitudinal fibers of the outer muscularis are now easily seen beneath the peritoneum. The rectum is usually not readily visible beneath the peritoneum, leading to the possibility of damage with thermal ablation.

scissors to minimize thermal damage. Arterial bleeds are coagulated with bipolar cautery; capillary bleeding will stop spontaneously. A rectal probe is useful. Once the nodule is outside the muscularis, the dissection is continued up to the vaginal wall. The nodule is then separated from the posterior wall of the uterus and from the vaginal wall. Since most recurrences are on the vaginal wall, one should remove all endometriosis on this site, and excision of part of the vaginal fornix may be needed. The vaginal opening is closed with two layers of running sutures using Monocryl 0.

7. Excision of the nodule from the sigmoid is facilitated by stabilizing the sigmoid with two

sutures to the round ligaments. Excision is done as for the rectum.

8. We rarely perform rectal resection, but are more liberal in performing it for the sigmoid colon. Only if the occlusion of the lumen is less than 50% for a length of less than 2.5 cm, we perform discoid excision. The nodule is usually located adjacent to and receiving its blood supply from the mesenterium. Dissection should start from this site, freeing the retraction and reducing vascularization. If the sigmoid becomes devascularized (as indicated by a change in color), then bowel resection is mandatory.

9. The next step is excision of the nodule from the vesico-uterine space. We recommend a ureteral stent if the nodule is larger than 1 cm. In the case of bladder resection, the bladder should be entered on the dome away from the ureters.

10. Hemostasis and repair of vagina, ureter, or bowel are performed if necessary.

11. Ovarian endometriosis is removed.

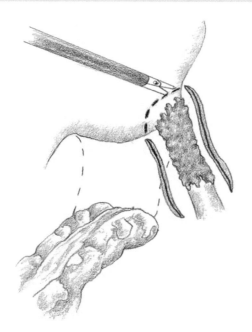

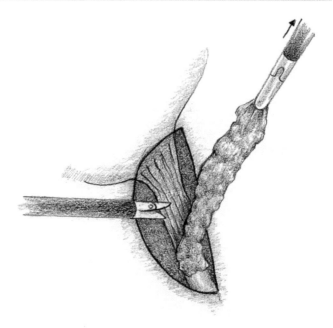

Figure 8.12 The right uterosacral ligament has been surrounded laterally and medially by lines of peritoneal incision. The uterosacral ligament will be transected at its insertion into the posterior cervix above the invasive disease using 50 W of coagulation current (dashed line).

Figure 8.14 Continued traction (straight arrow) allows the diseased portion of the ligament to be completely resected.

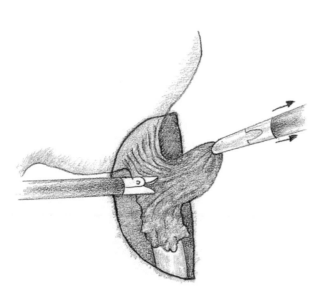

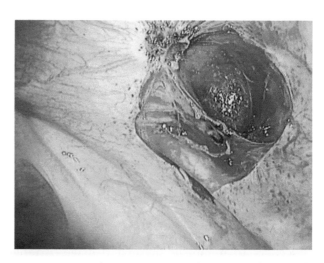

Figure 8.15 Endometriosis over the ureter that has been excised. (Courtesy of Togas Tulandi.)

Figure 8.13 Traction is used on the uterosacral ligament (straight arrows), while electrosurgery is used to shave the diseased tissue off the pelvic floor. Treatment of such invasive disease by thermal ablation would be problematic.

Complications and their prevention

- The bladder opening should be closed in two layers with a watertight suture, followed by insertion of an indwelling catheter for 7 days. Bladder atony can occur due to injury to the

parasympathetic nerves. Usually this recovers within 3–6 months.

- Ureter injury is repaired over a stent with one or two sutures of Monocryl 5-0. For ureter transection, we perform reanastomosis followed by an insertion of a ureteral stent. After repair of the ureter or the bladder, we routinely administer urinary antiseptics for 7 days.
- Even when carefully planned, surgery for adenomyotic nodules can be unpredictably difficult,

with its sequelae. A colorectal surgeon and an urologist should be consulted preoperatively.

- Rectal injury is closed with 3-0 Vicryl. For an opening of 3–5 cm, we place two lateral sutures and another on the middle. The opening is closed with two running sutures. The second-layer closure should incorporate the muscularis. A rectal probe can be useful to prevent strictures. It is also useful if the anatomy is distorted.
- Any defect on the muscularis layer of the bowel should be sutured. Some muscularis defects become visible only after the bowel is filled with 150 ml of a solution of methylene blue for the rectum and 350 ml for the sigmoid.
- When the bowel is opened, we irrigate the entire abdominal cavity liberally with 8 liters of saline. We leave a drain in the posterior cul-de-sac and another in the right paracolic gutter, and we administer antibiotics.
- Bowel perforation diagnosed after 48 hours requires a colostomy.
- Prolonged surgery increases the risks of compartment syndrome. If an operating time 5 hours is anticipated, excision of a nodule on the bladder or sigmoid nodule could be performed at future intervention. Alternatively, one can perform a laparotomy.

ACKNOWLEDGMENTS

I thank my collaborators, especially Mr Stephen Kennedy and Mr Enda McVeigh (Nuffield Department of obstetrics and gynaecology, Radcliffe Hospital, University of Oxford, UK), Dressa Anastasia Ussia (Villa Giose, Crotone, Italy), Dr Ornella Sizzi and Dr Alfonso Rosetti (Villa Valeria, Roma, Italy), and Dr Fiorenzo De Cicco (Universita del Sacro Cuore, Gemelli Hospitals, Roma, Italy). I thank my co-workers Dr Carlo De Cicco, Dr Juan Manuel de la Vega, Dr Lorena Ret Davalos, Dr John Koninckx, and Dr Jasper Verguts.

SUGGESTED READING

- Marcoux S, Maheux R, Berube S. Laparoscopic surgery in infertile women with minimal or mild endometriosis. Canadian Collaborative Group on Endometriosis. N Engl J Med 1997;337:217–22.
- Brosens IA, Van Ballaer P, Puttemans P, Deprest J. Reconstruction of the ovary containing large endometriomas by an extraovarian endosurgical technique. Fertil Steril 1996;66:517–21.
- Canis M, Pouly JL, Tamburro S, et al. Ovarian response during IVF-embryo transfer cycles after laparoscopic ovarian cystectomy for endometriotic cysts of >3 cm in diameter. Hum Reprod 2001; 16:2583–6.
- Chapron C, Chopin N, Borghese B, et al. Deeply infiltrating endometriosis: pathogenetic implications of the anatomical distribution. Hum Reprod 2006;21:1839–45.
- Koninckx PR, Martin DC. Surgical treatment of deeply infiltrating endometriosis. In: Sutton C, ed. Gynecological Endoscopic Surgery. London: Chapman and Hall, 1997: 19–35.
- Ret Davalos ML, De Cicco C, D'Hoore A, De Decker B, Koninckx PR. Outcome after rectum or sigmoid resection: a review for gynecologists. J Minim Invasive Gynecol 2007;14:33–38.

9

Laparoscopic treatment of polycystic ovarian syndrome

Togas Tulandi

The forerunner of laparoscopic treatment of polycystic ovarian syndrome (PCOS: Figure 9.1) is ovarian wedge resection by laparotomy. However, ovarian resection, whether performed by laparoscopy or by laparotomy, is associated with periadnexal adhesions and substantial tissue loss. Indeed, instances of premature ovarian failure have been described, rendering the procedure obsolete.

A less invasive procedure is laparoscopic ovarian drilling. This procedure is associated with restoration of menstruation and ovulation in 80% of cases. The pregnancy rates in clomiphene-resistant women are 36%, 54%, 68%, and 82% at 6, 12, 18, and 24 months of follow-up, respectively.

Recent studies have shown that metformin is equally efficacious as ovarian drilling. In addition, the advantages of metformin continue beyond conception. It reduces the miscarriage rate and decreases the likelihood of developing gestational diabetes. Our management strategy is to advocate weight loss followed by a trial of treatment with metformin alone and in combination with ovulation-inducing agents. Today, we rarely perform laparoscopic ovarian drilling. If, however, it is to be performed, the surgeon should carefully follow the procedure described below.

PROCEDURE

Unipolar needle electrodes and lasers are the tools used to perform ovarian drilling. However, the use of an insulated unipolar needle electrode is associated with less adhesion formation and a higher pregnancy rate than the use of a laser. As most of the uninsulated part of the needle is inside the ovary, this reduces the risk of electrical sparking and injury to intraabdominal organs.

The needle is inserted as perpendicular as possible to the ovarian surface. We use a short duration of cutting current of 100 W to assist entry of the needle. The surgeon inserts the whole length of the needle (8 mm) into the ovary, and ovarian drilling is performed using 40 W of coagulating current for 2 seconds at each point. The anterior surface is exposed by 'flipping' the ovary upward with forceps (Figure 9.2). Depending upon the size of the ovary, we create 10–15 punctures in each ovary (Figure 9.3). Liberal irrigation of the pelvic cavity to remove

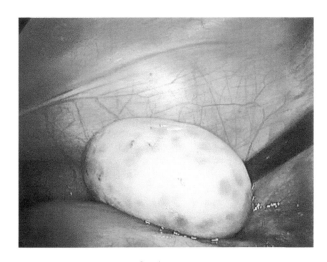

Figure 9.1 Appearance of polycystic ovaries.

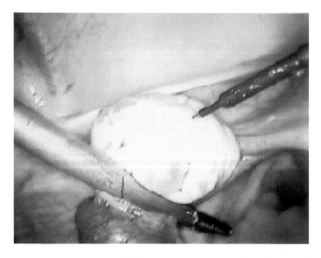

Figure 9.2 Ovarian drilling using an insulated unipolar needle electrode.

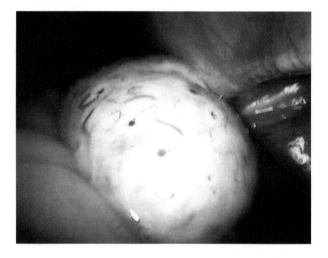

Figure 9.3 Appearance of the ovary after ovarian drilling.

necrotic debris and carbon materials is performed at completion of the procedure.

COMPLICATIONS AND THEIR PREVENTION

Excessive drilling may cause ovarian atrophy and premature menopause. Creating more than 20 craters per ovary and drilling the ovarian hilum should be avoided. This may jeopardize the blood supply to the ovary and may cause bleeding. Damage to the ovarian surface can cause periovarian adhesion which may further decrease fertility. Accordingly, the needle electrode should be inserted perpendicular to the ovarian surface until its insulated part is inside the ovary.

This procedure should be limited to clomiphene-resistant women who have failed metformin treatment and for some reason cannot be treated with gonadotropin, and to those who refuse to be treated with either in vitro fertilization or an in vitro maturation technique.

SUGGESTED READING

- Felemban A, Tan SL, Tulandi T. Laparoscopic treatment of polycystic ovaries with insulated needle cautery: a reappraisal. Fertil Steril 2000:73:266–9.
- Pirwany I, Tulandi T. Laparoscopic treatment of polycystic ovaries: Is it time to relinquish the procedure? Fertil Steril 2003;80:241–51.
- Al-Fadhli R, Tulandi T. Laparoscopic treatment of polycystic ovaries. Is its place diminishing? Curr Opin Obstet Gynecol 2004;16:295–8.

10

Laparoscopic preservation of female fertility

Togas Tulandi

Advances in cancer treatment have improved the long-term survival of young women suffering from malignancies. However, cancer therapies carry adverse effects, including loss of ovarian function and sterility. There have been a few options for young women undergoing cancer treatment, and the advent of new methods for preserving gonadal function and fertility is promising. Today, we can cryopreserve embryos, oocytes, and ovarian tissue, and in those undergoing pelvic irradiation, the physician should consider performing laparoscopic ovarian suspension.

LAPAROSCOPIC OVARIAN SUSPENSION

In women undergoing pelvic irradiation, the surgeon can move the ovaries out of the radiation field to avoid direct effects of ionizing radiation – a procedure called ovarian suspension, ovarian transposition, or oophoropexy. In women less than 40 years old, this is associated with preservation of ovarian function in 88.6% of cases. Concomitant excision of ovarian tissue for cryopreservation can be performed in the same setting.

Procedure (Figures 10.1–10.4)

To facilitate relocation of the ovaries above the pelvic brim, we use three trocars: the primary trocar is inserted 2 cm above the umbilicus and two secondary trocars at the same level. Following a thorough examination of the abdominal cavity, including the liver and diaphragm, the surgeon should perform a peritoneal washing for cytologic examination. The course of the ureter is followed; then the ovarian ligament is electrocoagulated and transected. Dissection is continued on the mesovarium until the infundibulopelvic ligament, but the vascular pedicle inside the ligament is left intact (Figures 10.2–10.5).

The ovary is mobilized superior and laterally to a new location above the pelvic brim. If mobilization is inadequate, the surgeon could perform a relaxing incision on the peritoneum inferior to the ovary. In our experience, we do not have to transect the tubes. This helps future spontaneous conception. The ovaries are sutured to the peritoneum with two sutures of 4-0 polydioxanone. At completion of the transposition, the ovary is marked with a metal clip. This is to facilitate future location of the ovaries by ultrasound or other imaging techniques.

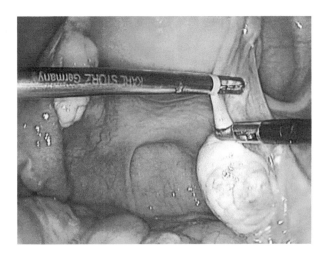

Figure 10.1 Laparoscopic ovarian transposition. The right ovarian ligament is being coagulated.

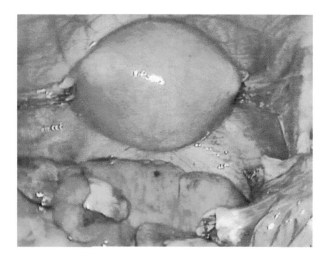

Figure 10.2 In this case, both ovarian ligaments and proximal fallopian tubes have been separated from the uterus.

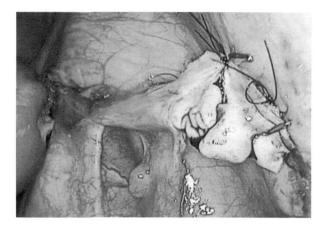

Figure 10.3 The right ovary has been transposed above the pelvic brim. Hemoclips have been placed on the ovary.

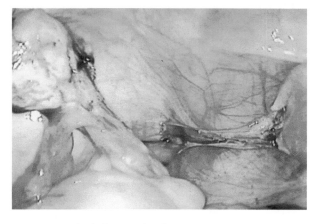

Figure 10.4 The left ovary has been transposed.

OVARIAN CRYOPRESERVATION

Ovarian cryopreservation is a new method to preserve fertility.

Procedure (Figure 10.5)

Laparoscopy excision of ovarian tissue for cryopreservation

The technique depends on how much ovarian tissue is to be excised. If one knows that the treatment will make the patient menopausal, it is logical to remove both ovaries. However, the psychological aspect of removal of both ovaries should be taken into account. Currently, we excise about only half of the ovary (Figure 10.5(a) and (b)). When the treating oncologist feels strongly that the patient will become menopausal, we remove one whole ovary. A few days before surgery, the embryologist should ascertain that the cryoprotective solution is available and not expired, and that he or she will be available to retrieve the specimen on removal.

The technique is performed by excising a portion of the ovary using laparoscopic scissors. Because of thermal damage to the ovarian tissue, the surgeon should not use electrocoagulation. The excised specimen is left attached to the ovary until the embryologist is ready to receive it. The tissue is removed from the abdominal cavity through a 10 mm port. We suture the ovarian opening using a few interrupted sutures of 4-0 polydioxanone. A small piece of ovarian tissue is sent for histopathologic examination. In those undergoing irradiation, the surgeon could perform both ovarian resection and laparoscopic ovarian transposition at the same setting.

Laparoscopic ovarian tissue transplantation

Several techniques have been described. One of the techniques involves transplanting frozen thawed ovarian tissue into an opening in the cortex of an ovary. The ovarian opening is then closed with 6-0 polyglactin sutures. One can also transplant the ovarian tissue by anchoring the tissue on the peritoneum of the ovarian fossa with sutures. A better method is to transplant the tissue in the peritoneal pocket in the ovarian fossa (Chapter 11).

(a)

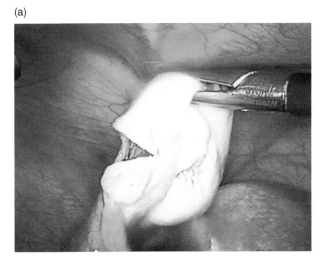

(b)

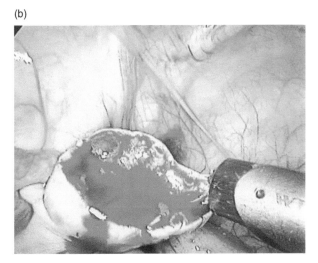

Figure 10.5 (a,b) Laparoscopic ovarian resection for cryopreservation: excision of one-third to a half of the ovary.

COMPLICATIONS AND THEIR PREVENTION

- The transposed ovary might slip back into the pelvic cavity. Accordingly, the surgeon should anchor it to the peritoneum with suture.
- The transplanted ovary might harbor malignant cells. Histopathologic examination of a piece of the ovarian tissue should be performed.

CONTRAINDICATIONS

Due to the possibility of developing cancer, one should not transplant ovaries from women with breast cancer.

SUGGESTED READING

- Tulandi T, Gosden R. Preservation of Fertility. London: Taylor & Francis, 2004:83–5.
- Bisharah M, Tulandi T. Laparoscopic preservation of ovarian function: an underused procedure. Am J Obstet Gynecol 2003;188:367–70.
- Donnez J, Dolmans MM, Demylle D, et al. Livebirth after orthotopic transplantation of cryopreserved ovarian tissue. Lancet 2004;364:1405–10.
- Radford JA, Lieberman BA, Brison D, et al. Orthotopic reimplantation of cryopreserved ovarian cortical strips after high-dose chemotherapy for Hodgkin's lymphoma. Lancet 2001;357:1172–5.
- Oktay K, Buyuk E, Veeck L, et al. Embryo development after heterotopic transplantation of cryopreserved ovarian tissue. Lancet 2004;363: 837–40.

11

Laparoscopic ovarian cryopreservation and reimplantation

Jacques Donnez, Marie-Madeleine Dolmans, Belen Martinez-Madrid, and Pascale Jadoul

Treatment of childhood and adult cancer with potentially sterilizing radiotherapy and/or chemotherapy may result in premature ovarian failure. Besides embryo and oocyte freezing, cryopreservation of ovarian tissue before cancer treatment is now a potential alternative for safeguarding fertility in women at risk of premature menopause.

Ovarian cryopreservation and transplantation procedures have so far been almost exclusively limited to avascular cortical fragments. In 2004, we reported the first live birth after ovarian cortex cryopreservation and reimplantation. In the case of ovarian cortex transplantation, small cortical pieces are grafted without vascular anastomosis and are completely dependent on the establishment of neovascularization after grafting. Consequently, the cells in the graft undergo significant ischemic and reperfusion damage, which can induce a high rate of follicular loss. Therefore, reducing the ischemic interval between transplantation and revascularization is essential to maintaining the viability and function of the graft. The best way to achieve this would be by transplantation of an intact ovary with vascular anastomosis, allowing immediate revascularization of the transplant.

PROCEDURE

Cryopreservation and reimplantation of ovarian cortex

Laparoscopic ovarian biopsy for cryopreservation

A laparoscopy is performed in the usual fashion. Ovarian biopsies are taken either with Palmer forceps, or with laparoscopic scissors. The size of the biopsies is determined by the chemotherapeutic or radiotherapeutic regimen to be administered. Premature ovarian failure after chemotherapy is dependent on age and the drug used and dose given, and does not occur in all cases. When there is a chance of recovery of ovarian function after treatment, we take two biopsies – about 12–15 mm long and 5 mm wide – from each ovary. When radiotherapy is indicated, the risk of premature ovarian failure is great and oophorectomy may be proposed. In the case of localized radiotherapy, ovarian transposition can be considered (Chapter 10).

Reimplantation of frozen-thawed ovarian tissue

- We perform the first laparoscopy 7 days before reimplantation to create a large peritoneal window just beneath the right ovarian hilus, followed by coagulation of the edges of the window (Figure 11.1). The goal was to induce angiogenesis and neovascularization in this area. We have recently modify our technique by excising the remaining ovarian cortex of the atrophic ovary and suturing pieces of frozen thawed ovarian cortex to the ovarian medulla with non-absorbable sutures (7.0 Prolene) (Figure 11.2). This procedure has the advantage of not requiring a first laparoscopy to induce neovascularization.

- At the second laparoscopy, we reimplant the thawed ovarian tissue. At the same time, biopsy samples 4–5 mm in size are taken from each of the atrophic ovaries to check for the presence of primordial follicles. We place the large strip and 35 small cubes of frozen–thawed ovarian tissue

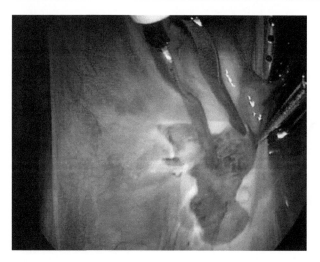

Figure 11.1 During the first laparoscopy (7 days before transplantation), a peritoneal window is created and the edges of the window are coagulated.

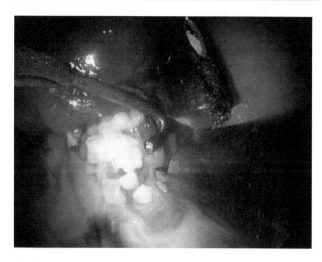

Figure 11.3 Large strips and small cubes of frozen–thawed ovarian tissue are placed into the furrow created by the peritoneal window very close to the ovarian vessels and fimbria.

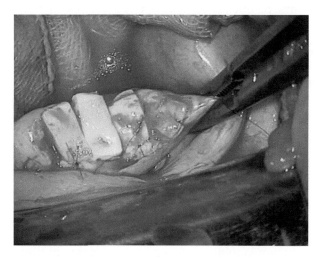

Figure 11.2 Ovarian cortical pieces measuring 4–5 mm to 1 cm in size are grafted onto the remaining ovary after the cortex of this ovary has been removed. Cortical pieces are sutured with 7-0 stitches.

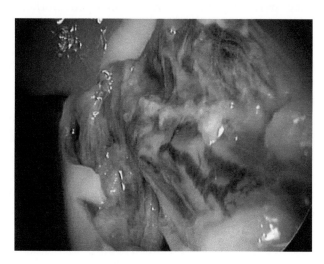

Figure 11.4 An extensive vascular network is clearly visible.

into a furrow created by the peritoneal window very close to the ovarian vessels and fimbria on the right side (Figure 11.3). No suture is used. An extensive neovascular network is clearly visible in this space (Figure 11.4).

- We also perform a third laparoscopy. The purpose is (1) to evaluate the viability of the orthotopic grafts 4 months after transplantation, by laparoscopic visualization and histologic analysis; (2) to check for the absence of any cellular growth anomalies (peritoneal fluid, histology), the cortical strip and cubes having been biopsied before

chemotherapy; (3) to reimplant the remaining ovarian cortical cubes at the patient's request.

Laparoscopic ovariectomy for whole-ovary cryopreservation and transplantation

To date, we have cryopreserved the entire ovary in nine patients.

Laparoscopic oophorectomy

Oophorectomy is performed in the standard fashion. However, bipolar coagulation is used sparingly. After dissection of the ureter, the posterior part of the broad ligament is opened with scissors (Figure 11.5). The ovarian pedicle and the ureter are dissected

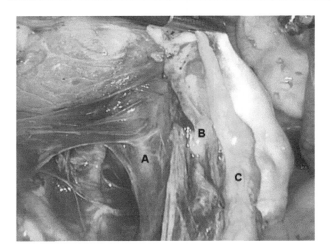

Figure 11.5 The broad ligament is opened between the infundibulopelvic ligament and the round ligament (A, ureter; B, ovarian pedicle, C, fallopian tube).

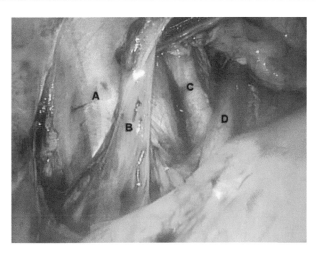

Figure 11.6 The ovarian pedicle is dissected cranially as high as possible, above the iliac vessels and psoas muscle (A, psoas muscle; B, ovarian pedicle; C, left iliac artery; D, ureter).

cranially as high as possible, above the iliac vessels and psoas muscle (Figure 11.6). An endoscopic pouch is introduced through the inferior medial trocar and opened in the pouch of Douglas.

The proximal isthmic part of the fallopian tube and the utero-ovarian ligament are clamped using two vascular clips and cut. The ovarian pedicle is then clamped using three vascular clips and cut between the two proximal clips (Figure 11.7). Care is always taken to place the clips as high as possible on the pedicle, leaving more than 5–6 cm of the vascular pedicle attached to the ovary. The freed ovary and fallopian tube are immediately placed in an endoscopic pouch and removed from the abdomen through the medial suprapubic incision, which is slightly enlarged to avoid damage to the ovary. The removed ovary is then immediately handed over to a second team present in the operating room, including a microsurgeon and biologist for perfusion and cryopreservation (Figure 11.8).

COMPLICATIONS AND THEIR PREVENTION

- The advantage of vascular transplants over avascular grafts of ovarian cortex is the decreased risk of ischemia and subsequent loss of primordial follicles.
- For oophorectomy and whole-ovary cryopreservation, the ovarian pedicle must be long enough to allow the ovarian artery and veins to be individualized and sutured to vessels of similar

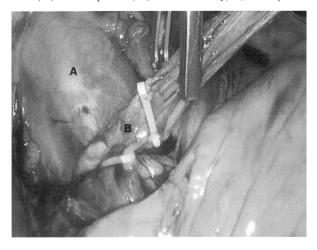

Figure 11.7 The ovarian pedicle is clamped using three vascular clips (A, psoas muscle; B, clipped ovarian pedicle).

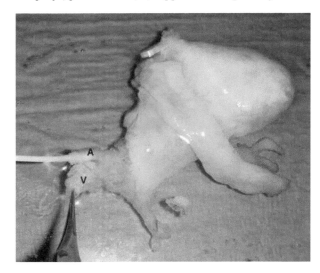

Figure 11.8 In the operating room, the ovarian artery (A) is catheterized under operative microscopic control and perfused. Liquid outflow allows identification of the ovarian veins (V) and their further microdissection.

diameter. In addition, the ischemic interval before cryopreservation must be as short as possible to avoid damage to the ovary.

- Ligation of the utero-ovarian ligament and the ovarian pedicle with five vascular clips is simpler and faster than using five sutures. This reduces the ischemic interval before ovarian artery perfusion with heparinized solution and cryoprotective medium.
- To reduce the ischemic period, the ovary should be immediately removed from the abdomen using an endoscopic pouch, which minimizes damage to the ovary. The endoscopic pouch should be properly placed in the abdominal cavity before the ovarian pedicle is clipped.
- A cooled sterile table equipped with a stereomicroscope and microsurgical instruments must be within easy reach, and the heparinized solution and cryoprotective medium ready for immediate use.

- Reimplantation of the ovary is contraindicated if there is a risk of neoplastic cell contamination in the ovary.

SUGGESTED READING

- Donnez J, Martinez-Madrid P, Jadoul P, et al. Ovarian tissue cryopreservation and existing alternatives: a review. Hum Reprod Update 2006;12:519–35.
- Donnez J, Dolmans MM, Demylle D, et al. Livebirth after orthotopic transplantation of cryopreserved ovarian tissue. Lancet 2004;364:1405–10.
- Jadoul P, Donnez J, Dolmans MM, et al. Laparoscopic ovariectomy for whole human ovary cryopreservation: technical aspects. Fertil Steril 2007; 87:971–5.
- Martinez-Madrid B, Dolmans MM, Van Langendonckt A, Defrere S, Donnez J. Freeze–thawing intact human ovary with its vascular pedicle with a passive cooling device. Fertil Steril 2004;82:1390–4.

12

Laparoscopic presacral neurectomy

Errico Zupi, Stefano Palomba, and Fulvio Zullo

The procedures described for the management of medically untreatable pelvic pain are classified as conservative or nonconservative. Conservative approaches includes pelvic denervations such as presacral neurectomy (PSN). This procedure, in addition to surgical treatment of endometriosis, is associated with a significant reduction in dysmenorrhea and in dyspareunia. We consider performing PSN only for chronic, intractable, and severe pelvic pain with midline component, that is of at least 6 months' duration, and that significantly reduces quality of life. Symptom relief is expected to last for at least 24 months after surgery. Careful selection of patients is crucial.

PROCEDURE

PSN involves total transection of the presacral nerves lying within the boundaries of the interiliac triangle. This area is defined caudally by the sacral promontory and laterally by the common iliac arteries meeting at the aortic bifurcation above (Figure 12.1).

- The first step is retraction of the sigmoid colon and identification of the major vessels (aortic bifurcation, bilateral common iliac arteries, inferior mesentery artery, and superior hemorrhoidal vessels). The sacral promontory area is infiltrated with vasoconstrictive solution to reduce blood loss. In order to have access to the retroperitoneal space, the peritoneum overlying the sacral promontory is elevated about 1 cm caudally to the aortic bifurcation and incised transversally. The peritoneum is dissected off the major vessels and the ureter on the right to the mesentery of the sigmoid colon on the left (Figure 12.2).

- The dissection on the retroperitoneum is extended caudally (Figure 12.3). The excised edges of the presacral area are cauterized using bipolar forceps and the presacral area is exposed with blunt dissection of the underlying adipose tissues. To reduce bleeding, the blunt dissection is performed transversally, avoiding major vessels. Bleeding is generally controlled with the use of electrocautery. A semilunar piece of retroperitoneal tissue is excised and sent for pathologic confirmation of nerve fibers.

- Adjacent to the aortic bifurcation, two or three large continuous nerve bundles will constitute the superior hypogastric plexus. In the area more caudal to the sacral promontory, the nerve fibers are less distinct and 12–15 individual fibers will be present. All underlying tissue layers down to the periosteum are cauterized and resected. At the end of the procedure, all the presacral nerves lying within the boundaries of the interiliac triangle should be totally removed or destroyed (Figure 12.4).

COMPLICATIONS AND THEIR PREVENTION

Intraoperative complications

- Despite the operative field being in close proximity to large vessels and the right ureter, major

(a)

(b)

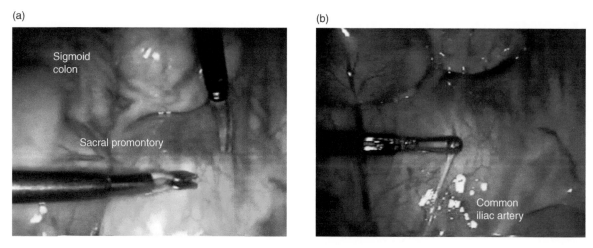

Figure 12.1 (a, b) The presacral area (the interiliac triangle). After retraction of the sigmoid colon, it is possible to observe caudally the sacral promontory and laterally the common iliac arteries meeting at the aortic bifurcation above.

(a)

(b)

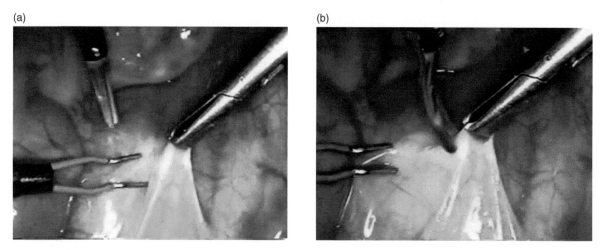

Figure 12.2 After infiltration of the sacral promontory with vasoconstrictive solution, access to the retroperitoneal space is obtained, elevating the peritoneum overlying the sacral promontory (a) and incising it transversally (b).

(a)

(b)

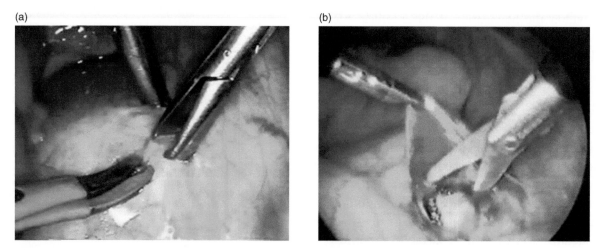

Figure 12.3 The peritoneal incision is extended caudally. The excised edges are coagulated (a) and the presacral area is exposed with blunt dissection of the underlying adipose tissues (b).

(a)

(b)

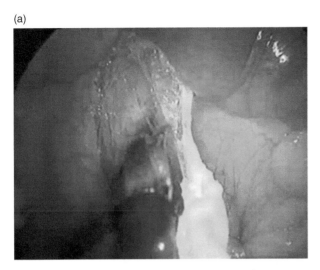 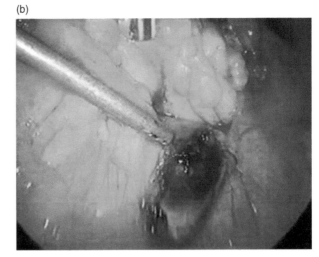

Figure 12.4 (a, b) All underlying tissue down to the periosteum of the sacral area is totally removed or destroyed.

intraoperative complications are rare. The incidence of injury to major vessels is extremely low (0.15%).

- The most common serious intraoperative complication is sacral hemorrhage. Although the middle sacral vein should be routinely identified and isolated, several branches of the presacral venous plexus could be lacerated during blunt dissection of the presacral area. The valveless intrasacral venous plexus has extensive collateral venous circulation and numerous perforating vessels that exit into the anterior sacrum. Bleeding can usually be electrocoagulated, but it is sometimes necessary to use suture ligation or hemoclips. Rarely, placing of stainless steel thumbtacks into each foramen is needed.
- Another rare intraoperative complication is damage to presacral lymphatic vessels or plexus, with leakage of milky chyle. In our experience, using bipolar forceps for dissection of the presacral area, we have never encountered injury of lymphatic vessels with chylous ascites. Most chylous ascites has been observed after using unipolar scissors. The treatment is similar to that of injury to the middle sacral veins (bipolar coagulation, suture ligation, hemoclips, or stainless steel thumbtacks). Possible chylostasis should be examined under low peritoneal pneumatic pressure. In the presence of chylostasis, one should place a drain inside the pelvic cavity. The drain can be removed after no further chylous drainage is observed.

- In most cases, injury to the lymphatic system is not recognized during surgery. Patients may experience progressive abdominal distention, abdominal tenderness, and rebound pain a few days after the surgery. The diagnosis is made by the findings of milky fluid at culdocentesis or paracentesis. In mild cases, treatment consists of percutaneous drainage, bed rest, and a high-protein, low-fat, medium-chain triglyceride diet to decrease chyle production.
- Particular attention should be paid to electrolyte imbalance, hypoproteinemia, and risk of infection. If this treatment fails, a laparoscopy to exclude injury of the large lymphatic vessels or other vital organs should be done. However, it is rare to identify and seal single lymphatic vessels. During laparoscopy, the excised edges of the presacral area should be coagulated and the peritoneum over the presacral area sutured.

Postoperative complications

Because of potential damage related to innervation of the colon and bladder, patients affected by or with a history of severe constipation and/or urinary retention should be carefully informed of the potential long-term complications of this surgical procedure.

- Immediate postoperative complications include transient hypotension, and urinary retention. About 1–10% of patients experience urinary urgency a few days after surgery. Although spontaneous improvement has been noted, the improvement has been minimal even with medical treatment.
- The most common complication of PSN is bowel dysfunction especially constipation, in 4–74% of cases.
- Labor dysfunction and vaginal dryness are reported by 2–3% of patients.

SUGGESTED READING

- Steege JF. Presacral neurectomy. In: Nichols DH, Clarke-Pearson DL, eds. Gynecologic, Obstetric, and Related Surgery, 2nd edn. St Louis, MO: Mosby, 2000.

- Palomba S, Zullo F. Pelvic denervations procedures as surgical management of pelvic pain due to endometriosis. In: Sutton C, Jones KD, Adamson GD, eds. Modern Management of Endometriosis. London: Taylor & Francis, 2005:139–51.
- Zullo F, Palomba S, Zupi E, *et al*. Effectiveness of presacral neurectomy in women with severe dysmenorrhea caused by endometriosis who were treated with laparoscopic conservative surgery: a 1-year prospective randomized double-blind controlled trial. Am J Obstet Gynecol 2003;189: 5–10.
- Zullo F, Palomba S, Zupi E, *et al*. Long-term effectiveness of presacral neurectomy for the treatment of severe dysmenorrhea due to endometriosis. J Am Assoc Gynecol Laparosc 2004;11:23–8.
- Nezhat CH, Seidman DS, Nezhat FR, *et al*. Long-term outcome of laparoscopic presacral neurectomy for the treatment of central pelvic pain attributed to endometriosis. Obstet Gynecol 1998; 91:701–4.

13

Laparoscopic myomectomy and laparoscopic uterine artery occlusion

Charles E Miller and Moises Lichtinger

Laparoscopic myomectomy continues to have an important place in the gynecologic surgery. This is especially true for women of reproductive age. With advances in laparoscopic suturing technique and instrumentation, most myomectomies can be performed via the laparoscope. The results are comparable to those of myomectomy by laparotomy. Moreover, the procedure is associated with faster recovery, and less adhesion formation.

Laparoscopic uterine artery occlusion is another surgical option for patients with symptomatic leiomyomas. It produces transient uterine ischemia and subsequent relief of leiomyoma symptoms. It can be performed simultaneously with laparoscopic myomectomy to reduce intraoperative bleeding and facilitate uterine reconstruction. This procedure is for patients with symptomatic leiomyomas with perfused intramural fibroids. Those with no fibroid perfusion (calcified, degeneration), or submucous or subserosal location and those who have had uterine artery embolization are not candidates for laparoscopic uterine artery occlusion. Pedunculated fibroids are best treated with myomectomy.

PREOPERATIVE EVALUATION

Because the laparoscopy does not provide the same tactile feedback as an open procedure, in order to perform successful laparoscopic myomectomy, the exact number, location, and site of the uterine myomata must be known before surgery. We perform a three-dimensional sonohysterogram prior to all myomectomy procedures. When the uterus is large, transabdominal ultrasound or magnetic resonance imaging (MRI) is recommended.

We perform an endometrial biopsy in all women over the age of 40. If the patient is anemic, a gonadotropin-releasing hormone (GnRH) agonist can be utilized for 3 months to promote amenorrhea and to improve the hematologic status of the patient.

PROCEDURE FOR LAPAROSCOPIC MYOMECTOMY

It is important to understand the various concepts involved that will make laparoscopic myomectomy efficient and safe. The ultimate test of the procedure is the occurrence of a pregnancy and its outcome.

1. The patient is prepared for the laparoscopic procedure in a standard manner. We routinely perform hysteroscopy to rule out and to remove undiagnosed submucous fibroid. An intrauterine manipulator is then inserted. Good uterine manipulation can be achieved by placing a sufficiently long manipulator that reaches the uterine fundus.
2. The trocars must be placed higher than the uterus. If the uterus is large, one should consider placing the first trocar above the umbilicus. Similarly, the secondary trocars are placed lateral and higher than the mass.
3. Concomitant procedures such as lysis of adhesions or excision of endometriosis are completed before myomectomy.

4. We first infiltrate the myometrium surrounding the myoma with a dilute solution of vasopressin (30 units in 100 ml of saline). Before injecting, the plunger should be first aspirated to avoid intravascular injection of vasopressin. This part of the uterus blanches.

5. A vertical incision on the serosa and myometrium is performed. Compared with a horizontal incision, this type of incision facilitates repair using two lateral trocars. Once the cleavage plane is reached, the fibroid will protrude out (Figures 13.1–13.3). It is important to use energy that cuts with minimal tissue desiccation. We use the Harmonic Scalpel (Ethicon Endo-Surgery, Inc.). One can also use unipolar cautery. We remove multiple myomas through a single incision.

6. If the endometrial cavity is entered, we approximate the endometrium with simple interrupted sutures of 3-0 polydioxanone (PDS) 1–2 mm apart. The uterine incision is repaired in multiple layers. It is imperative that we eliminate the dead space to minimize hematoma formation and to maximize tissue repair. Depending on the defect shape and site, one can use an interrupted 'pursestring' suture, a 'mattress' suture, or a continuous suture with the same suture material to close the myometrium. The serosa is repaired separately using a 3-0 or 4-0 PDS suture with buried knots, mattress style, baseball style, or imbricating continuous closure.

7. Morcelation is performed after complete repair of the uterus. Occasionally, morcelation is done in situ midway through the myoma extraction to enable visualization. We use a 12 mm umbilical port for morcelation. Others use the lateral port (Figure 13.4).

8. At the completion of the procedure, we irrigate and perform meticulous hemostasis. We then place an anti-adhesive barrier.

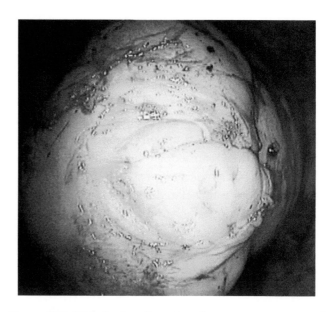

Figure 13.2 With further dissection, the myoma comes out of the uterine incision.

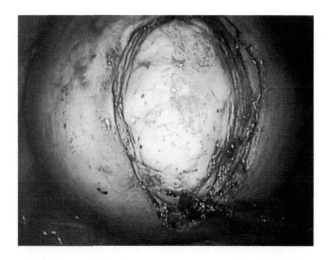

Figure 13.1 A vertical incision has been made on the uterine wall with a unipolar spatula. The myoma has started to come out of the uterine opening. (Courtesy of Togas Tulandi.)

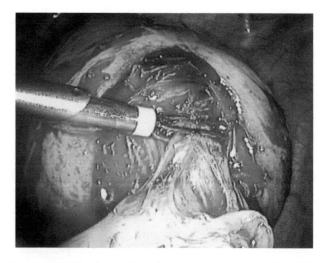

Figure 13.3 Blood vessels at the base of the myoma should be coagulated.

PROCEDURE FOR LAPAROSCOPIC UTERINE ARTERY OCCLUSION

1. The procedure starts by incising the peritoneum over the psoas muscle lateral to the broad ligament (Figure 13.5). This prevents injury to major retroperitoneal vessels, releases lateral displacement of the uterus by myomas, and allows entry into the retroperitoneal space.
2. The dissection is continued below the round ligament and lateral to the uterus anteriorly in the perivesical space. The obliterated lateral umbilical ligament is identified, traced cephalad, and pushed laterally at its entrance to the hypogastric artery (Figures 13.6 and 13.7). In this area, the origin of the uterine artery can be seen (Figure 13.8).
3. The first 2–3 cm of the uterine artery has a straight tract. Two vascular clips are applied on the uterine artery. Following occlusion of both arteries, blanching of the uterus can be seen (Figure 13.9).

COMPLICATIONS AND THEIR PREVENTION

- Complications related to laparoscopy in general include incisional hernia, pelvic infection, and pulmonary emboli.

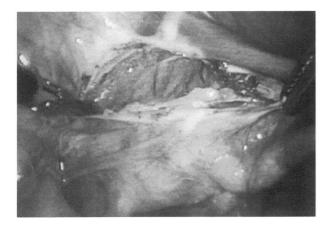

Figure 13.4 Morcellation of the myoma from the lateral trocar. (Courtesy of Togas Tulandi.)

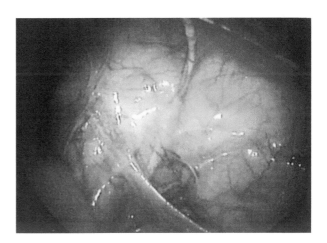

Figure 13.6 The obliterated umbilical artery becomes retroperitoneal as it passes under the round ligament.

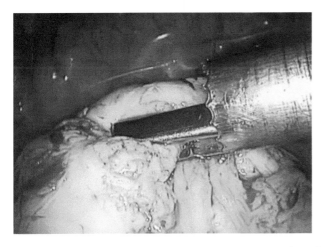

Figure 13.5 The right peritoneum is incised laterally next to the round ligament over the psoas muscle.

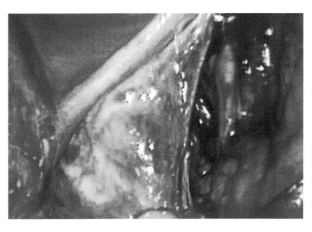

Figure 13.7 The fibrous white element (obliterated umbilical artery) ends at the internal iliac artery.

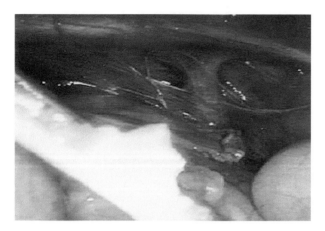

Figure 13.8 Proximal uterine artery.

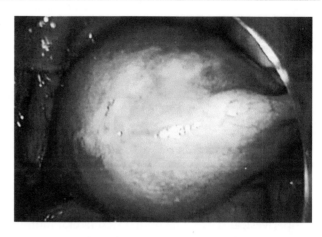

Figure 13.9 Bilateral uterine artery occlusion produces blanching of the uterus.

- Possible myomectomy complications are bleeding from the uterine incision and uterine rupture in pregnancy or in labor. Multilayered closure and meticulous hemostasis are mandatory. Only surgeons who are familiar with laparoscopic suturing should perform laparoscopic myomectomy.
- Complications of laparoscopic uterine occlusion are similar to those of uterine artery embolization. We believe that it is rarely needed and should be done only concomitant with myomectomy.

SUGGESTED READING

- Lichtinger M, Hallson L, Calvo P, Adeboyejo G. Laparoscopic uterine artery occlusion for symptomatic leiomyomas. J Am Assoc Gynecol Laparosc 2002;9:191–8.
- Burbank F, Hutchins FL Jr. Uterine artery occlusion by embolization or surgery for the treatment of fibroids: a unifying hypothesis – transient uterine ischemia. J Am Assoc Gynecol Laparosc 2000;7(4 Suppl):S1–49.
- Tulandi T. Treatment of uterine fibroids. Is surgery obsolete? N Engl J Med 2007;356:411–13.

14

Laparoscopic total and supracervical hysterectomy

Togas Tulandi

It is estimated that about 600 000 hysterectomies are performed annually in the USA, with the most common indications being uterine fibroids and abnormal uterine bleeding.

The purpose of the procedure is to reduce the morbidity that occurs with laparotomy. There are several types of laparoscopic hysterectomy. In 1982, Semm introduced laparoscopic-assisted vaginal hysterectomy (LAVH), where laparoscopy is used to visualize the abdomen, to remove adhesions, or to develop surgical planes followed by vaginal hysterectomy. In 1989, Reich first reported hysterectomy performed by laparoscopy. When the cervix is left in situ, it becomes a laparoscopic supracervical hysterectomy (LASH). A modification of LASH is classic intrafascial supracervical hysterectomy (CISH), where the endocervical canal is cored and removed. The latter is not widely performed.

Today, we perform LASH or laparoscopic total hysterectomy (LTH). For LASH, a morcellator should be available (Figure 14.1). The conduct of LTH is facilitated by the Rumy system (Figure 14.2). Because of the advantages of laparoscopy over laparotomy, in most cases a laparoscopic procedure is preferable to the abdominal approach. However, in those with a mobile uterus of <12 weeks' gestational size and some degree of uterine descent, vaginal hysterectomy should be considered.

LAPAROSCOPIC TOTAL HYSTERECTOMY

LTH is an operation in which the surgeon performs most or all steps of the procedure by laparoscopy.

Procedure

- We use a primary and two secondary trocars. They should be inserted higher than the upper margin of the uterus. A uterine manipulator is inserted for good manipulation of the uterus throughout the procedure.
- The course of the ureter should always be followed before and throughout the procedure. In order to facilitate continuous identification of the ureter, we open the peritoneum just above the ureter for about 1 cm length (Figure 14.3). Dissection above this marked point is considered safe.
- For ovarian removal, we secure the infundibulopelvic ligament with bipolar cautery and then transect. If the ovaries are to be retained, ligation and transection is performed on the ovarian ligaments.
- The same procedure is repeated on the round ligament. We separate the two leaves of the broad ligament, exposing the uterine vessels along the side of the uterus (Figure 14.4).
- The bladder flap is developed by cutting the bladder peritoneum between the cervix and the bladder with scissors. This is facilitated by hydrodissection using a solution of normal saline (Figure 14.5). The bladder is dissected off the lower uterine segment and the cervix until the endopelvic fascia overlying the cervix is identified. This frequently requires the use of an endoscopic swab ('peanut' gauze) (Figure 14.6).
- We coagulate the uterine vessels with bipolar cautery. Once the uterus is blanched, we transect

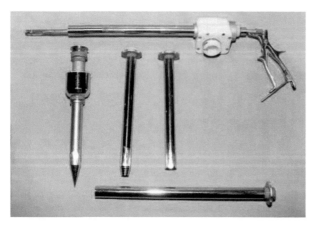

Figure 14.1 Morcellator for laparoscopic supracervical hysterectomy.

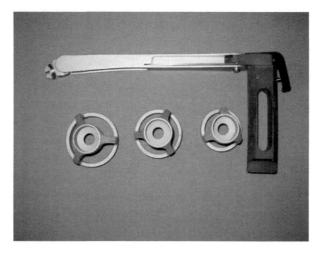

Figure 14.2 Rumy system for total laparoscopic hysterectomy.

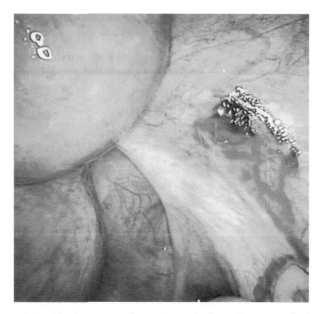

Figure 14.3 A peritoneal opening just above the ureter facilitates continuous identification of the ureter.

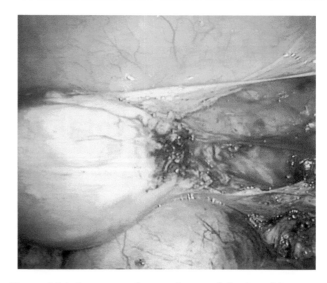

Figure 14.4 Separating the two leaves of the broad ligament exposes the right uterine vessels along the side of the uterus. Note a large ovarian cyst behind the uterus.

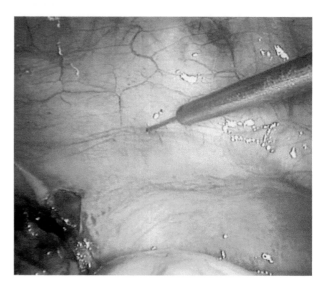

Figure 14.5 Hydrodissection of the bladder peritoneum by injecting normal saline solution.

the vessels, and then push them caudally until they reach below the cervix. In most cases, we also use hemoclips (Figure 14.7).

• The uterine manipulator is then replaced with a Rumy uterine manipulator with its cervical cup or a vaginal cylinder tube (Figure 14.8). It allows us to cut the vaginal wall circumferentially around the upper margin of the cup (Figure 14.9). By cutting the vaginal fornix very close to the cervix it decreases the risks of ureter injury. Loss of pneumoperitoneum is avoided by insufflating the vaginal balloon with 60 ml of saline solution.

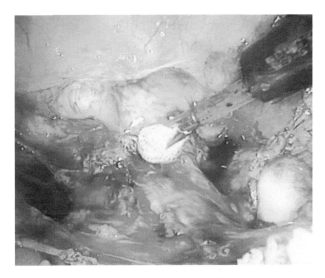

Figure 14.6 Dissection the bladder off the cervix using a 'peanut' gauze.

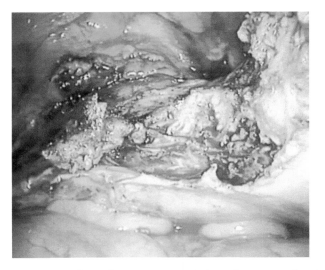

Figure 14.7 The right uterine vessels have been coagulated and secured with hemoclips.

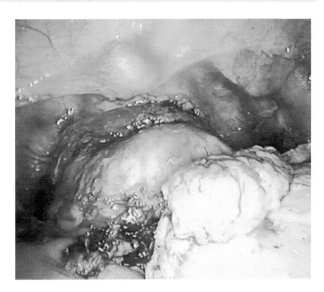

Figure 14.8 The cervical cup inside the vagina bulges the fornix.

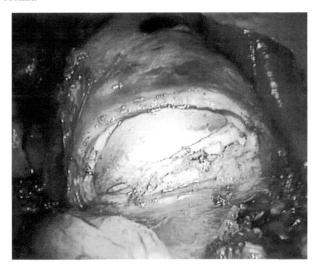

Figure 14.9 The vagina is cut circumferentially around the upper margin of the cup.

- The uterus and adnexa are delivered through the vaginal opening. Usually we leave the uterus in the vagina to prevent loss of carbon dioxide gas. Otherwise, we insert a glove filled with sponges into the vagina. A large uterus may need to be morcellated first.
- The vaginal opening is closed with three figure-of-eight sutures of polydioxanone (PDS 0 or 1 sutures) (Figure 14.10).
- At completion of the hysterectomy, we perform liberal peritoneal lavage. All pedicles are inspected and further hemostasis is performed if needed.

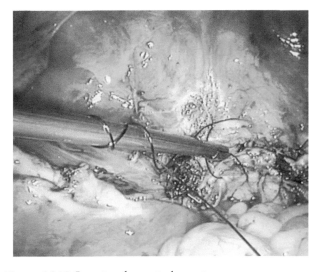

Figure 14.10 Suturing the vaginal opening.

LAPAROSCOPIC SUPRACERVICAL HYSTERECTOMY (LASH)

Supracervical or subtotal hysterectomy is defined as removal of the uterine corpus while leaving the cervix in place. This procedure is associated with rare urologic complications. LASH is appropriate for benign pathologic condition above the cervix, including uterine myomas, adenomyosis, or intractable abnormal uterine bleeding.

Procedure

- The procedure is performed in a similar fashion as for LTH. The uterine vessels are coagulated but not transected. After the uterus is blanched, we place an Endoloop (Edicon Endo-Surgery, Inc.) around the cervix (Figure 14.11). The uterine manipulator is removed and another Endoloop is placed. The cervix is then amputated with scissors, an ultrasonic scalpel, a unipolar electrode or a loop-electrode (Figure 14.12).

- The uterus is morcellated using a 2 cm electric morcellator inserted through one of the secondary trocars (Figure 14.13).
- In premenopausal women, at the completion of LASH, coagulation of the endocervical canal should be performed (Figure 14.14). This is to decrease the occurrence of cyclic bleeding.

POTENTIAL COMPLICATIONS AND THEIR PREVENTION

- In general, women with a uterus >16 weeks' gestational size and those with malignancies are

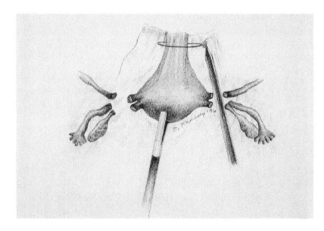

Figure 14.12 Laparoscopic subtotal hysterectomy: application of a pretied ligature (loop) after ligation of the uterine vessels.

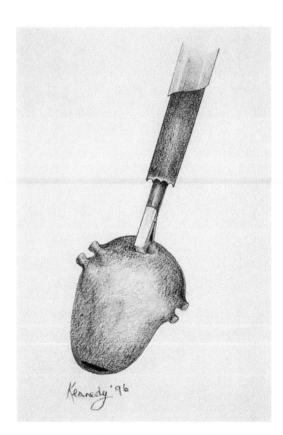

Figure 14.11 Morecellation of the Uterine Corpus.

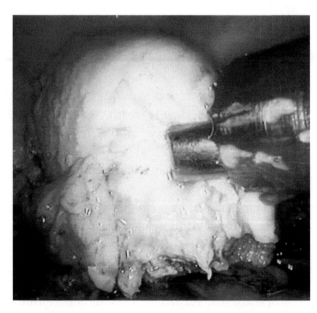

Figure 14.13 Morcellation of the uterine corpus.

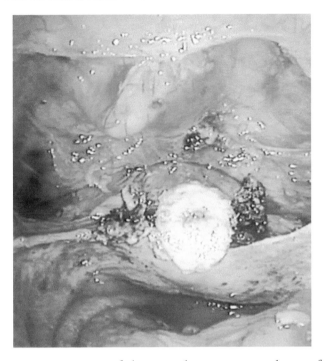

Figure 14.14 View of the cervical stump at completion of laparoscopic supracervical hysterectomy. The endocervix has been coagulated.

not candidates for laparoscopic hysterectomy. However, each surgeon might place an upper limit of the uterine size based on personal preference and expertise. Instead of uterine size, access to the uterine vessels dictates the feasibility of laparoscopic hysterectomy, and this can only be determined intraoperatively. The patient should be informed about the possibility of a laparotomy.

• The course of the ureter should be followed during the procedure. To avoid ureteral injury, the staple, if used, should not be placed below the uterine vessels.

• Instead of LASH, the hysterectomy of choice in women with abnormal cervical pathology is LTH.

• In premenopausal women, at the completion of LASH, coagulation of the endocervical canal should be performed. The incidences of cyclic bleeding with and without coagulation of the endocervical canal are 2.4% and 17%, respectively.

• The morcellator should be used cautiously. The operator should visualize its sharp end all the time. Accordingly, morcellation from one of the lateral trocars is preferable than through the primary umbilical port.

• Preoperatively, the patient should be warned about the possibility of complications, including bowel perforation, bladder or ureteral injury, as well as other possible complications of laparoscopy. In the postoperative period, observations of fever, urinary symptoms, abdominal distention, bowel habit, and abdominal pain are extremely important.

SUGGESTED READING

• Reich H, DeCaprio J, McGlynn F. Laparoscopic hysterectomy. J Gynecol Surg 1989;5:213–16.
• Garry R, Fountain J, Mason S, et al. The eVALuate study: two parallel randomized trials one comparing laparoscopic with abdominal hysterectomy, the other comparing laparoscopic with vaginal hysterectomy. BMJ 2004;328:129–33.
• Milad MP, Sokol E. Laparoscopic morcellator-related injuries. J Am Assoc Gynecol Laparosc 2003;10:383–5.
• McCartney AJ, Obermaier A. Total laparoscopic hysterectomy with a transvaginal tube. J Am Assoc Gynecol Laparosc 2004;11:79–82.

15

Laparoscopic radical hysterectomy

Konstantin Zakashansky and Farr Nezhat

The term 'radical hysterectomy' refers to *en bloc* excision of the uterus with the parametrial tissue, including the round, broad, cardinal, and uterosacral ligaments, and the upper one-third to one-half of the vagina.

Open radical hysterectomy has been the gold standard of care for the treatment of early stage cervical cancer for decades. However, recent advances in laparoscopic instrumentation have made it possible to safely perform radical hysterectomy laparoscopically. Whether the procedure is performed open or laparoscopically, a thorough knowledge of pelvic anatomy and meticulous attention to dissection are critical to avoid damage to the ureters, bladder and rectum. One of the major benefits of the laparoscopic approach is superior visualization due to pneumo distension and optical magnification. This enhanced visualization enables improved small blood vessel access and identification, which results in less blood loss, as well as unparalleled precision during the ureteric dissection. Other advantages of laparoscopic radical hysterectomy echo those seen with laparoscopy in general such as shorter hospitalization, faster bowel function recovery, less postoperative pain, and decreased overall cost.

The 5 year overall survival for patients with Stage IA2 or IB1 cancer following laparoscopic, just as with an open, radical hysterectomy is close to 96%.

PROCEDURE

- Standard *preoperative preparation* includes outpatient mechanical bowel evacuation and perioperative prophylactic antibiotics.
- Four trocars are placed as shown in Figure 15.1.
- *Exploration of the abdominal and pelvic cavity* is performed first. Prior to proceeding with a radical hysterectomy, any lesions that appear suspicious for malignancy are biopsied. The para-aortic lymph nodes are inspected first, followed by the pelvic lymph nodes. If gross para-aortic metastatic disease is present, radical hysterectomy is usually abandoned. Laparoscopic para-aortic lymph node dissection is performed in selected cases if microscopic disease is suspected and if frozen-section evaluation can be performed. Management of patients with malignant pelvic lymph nodes is controversial. We usually proceed with the radical hysterectomy in cases where the pelvic lymph nodes can be completely resected.
- Proceeding with a radical hysterectomy requires that *six avascular pelvic spaces be developed* and that the bladder and rectum be mobilized. Traditionally, we start out by dissecting the rectovaginal space. The uterus is sharply anteverted using uterine manipulation and the peritoneum between the uterosacral ligaments is incised using the harmonic shear in variable mode; the rectum can then be gently brought down away from the

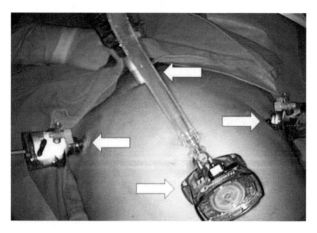

Figure 15.1 Four-trocar placement for total laparoscopic radical hysterectomy and bilateral pelvic lymphadenectomy. The arrows mark the locations of the trocars. A 5–10 mm trocar is placed at the umbilicus, a 5–10 mm trocar is placed in the suprapubic region, and two additional 5 mm trocars are placed bilaterally in the lower quadrants.

(a)

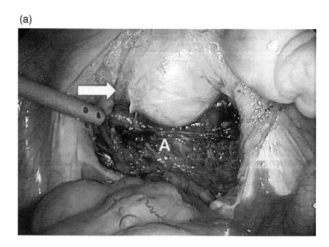

(b)

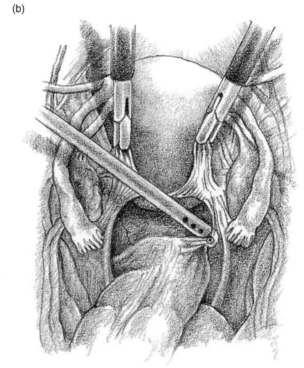

Figure 15.2 (a) Development of the rectovaginal space (A). The posterior vaginal fornix is placed on tension (marked by the arrow) and a moistened sponge on sponge-forceps is placed in the vagina to facilitate delineation of the tissue planes. (b) Diagram of complete development of the rectovaginal space.

vagina. A moistened sponge on a sponge-forceps is placed in the posterior vaginal fornix to facilitate visualization and development of this surgical plane (Figure 15.2).

- The surgeon subsequently begins the *pelvic wall dissection*. After round ligaments on either side of the uterus are coagulated and cut using harmonic shears or scissors, the anterior leaf of the broad ligament is opened bilaterally. The bladder flap is developed using both blunt and sharp dissection. The bladder is gradually dissected away from the cervix and vagina, and once again a moistened sponge on a sponge-forceps is placed in the anterior vaginal fornix to facilitate development of the vesicovaginal space (Figure 15.3).

- The posterior leaf of the broad ligament is opened, and the *paravaginal and pararectal spaces are developed* using gentle blunt dissection. If ovarian preservation is indicated or desired, the ovarian ligament and the proximal portion of the fallopian tube are coagulated and divided. If the adnexa are to be removed, the infundibulopelvic ligament is isolated, desiccated, and divided using the harmonic shears or LigaSure. The paravesical space is developed by placing tension on the umbilical ligaments, with blunt dissection being performed with the harmonic shears and suction irrigator. The dissection is continued inferiorly to the iliac vessels, after which the obturator space is

developed. The structures surrounding the obturator space, including the obturator internus muscle and pubic bone, are visualized and care is taken to avoid injury to the obturator nerve and vessels that traverse this area.

- After development of the paravesical and pararectal spaces, pelvic *lymphadenectomy* can be performed. This involves removal of the lymph node packets from the common iliac vessels and

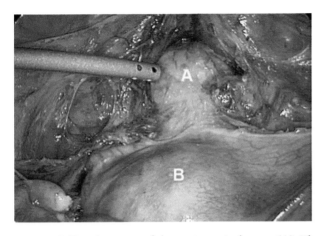

Figure 15.3 Development of the vesicovaginal space (A). The uterus (B) is pushed cephalad into the abdominal cavity to facilitate visualization.

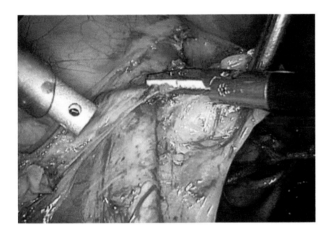

Figure 15.4 Left pelvic lymphadenectomy.

external iliac vessels down to the level of the deep circumflex veins (Figure 15.4). The obturator nerve is identified and the obturator fossa nodes and the hypogastric nodes are completely removed and sent for pathologic examination. At this point, the medial umbilical ligament is suspended with upward tension and the origin of the uterine artery from the hypogastric artery is identified.

- *The uterine artery is desiccated* and divided at its origin using endoscopic shears or LigaSure vessel sealant as shown in Figure 15.5. In a similar fashion, the uterine vein is also identified, desiccated, and cut. The uterine vessels are placed on medial tension and the ureter is unroofed. The curved tip of the harmonic shears is used to

dissect the ureter out of the tunnel (Figure 15.6). The parametrium is coagulated and then divided laterally (Figure 15.7); in this manner, the ureter is completely unroofed. The uterosacral ligaments, cardinal ligaments, and a portion of the paracolpos are then divided enabling complete mobilization of the uterus. Upon complete mobilization of the uterus, the laparoscopic portion of the procedure is temporarily suspended.

- Although we used to open and close the vagina endoscopically, we have since found the vaginal approach to be preferable because it allows for superior visualization and delineation of the vaginal margins. Thus, at this point in the surgery, the Humi uterine manipulator is removed and *the vagina is cut under direct visualization* around the cervix to ensure adequate margins. The hysterectomy specimen is removed and sent to pathology. The vaginal cuff is closed using 0 Vicryl sutures in a figure-of-eight fashion.

- After removal of the specimen and *closure of the vaginal cuff*, the pelvic cavity is thoroughly irrigated with normal saline (Figure 15.8). Once the surgeon has ensured hemostasis, indigo carmine is administered intravenously to assess for ureteral and bladder injury. The rectum is insufflated with air and is evaluated intraabdominally under saline to rule out injury to the bowel. The bladder is then distended with saline to further ensure its integrity.

- *Postoperatively*, early ambulation and oral intake are encouraged. Patients are usually discharged home on the second or third postoperative day with a Foley catheter in place. The catheter is removed, in the office, 7–10 days after surgery.

Contraindications

Absolute contraindications to the laparoscopic approach are any medical conditions that prevent appropriate anesthesia administration, positioning of the patient for surgery, or prolonged pneumoperitoneum, such as a severe restrictive lung disease, hip disease, or a ventriculo-peritoneal shunt. The following conditions are considered to be relative contraindications for laparoscopic hysterectomy, and should be considered on a case by case basis: a history of multiple prior abdominal surgeries with extensive

(a)

(b)

(c)

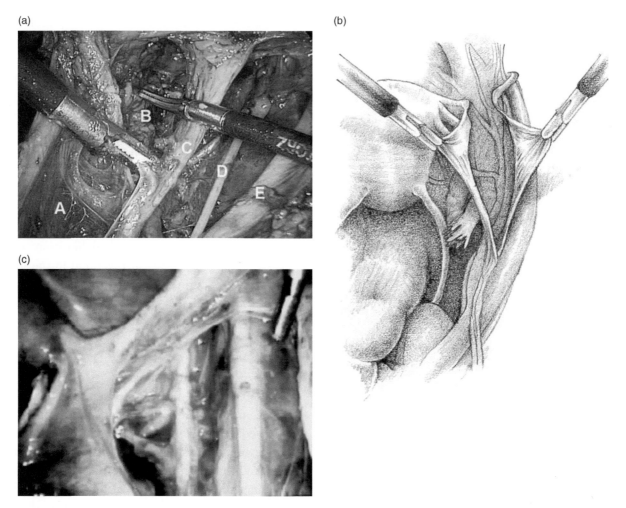

Figure 15.5 (a) Isolation, coagulation, and division of the right uterine artery at its origin using harmonic shears. The right pararectal (A) and paravesical (B) spaces have been fully developed; and the right umbilical artery (C), right obturator nerve (D), and right external iliac vein (E) are visible. (b) Exposing the paravesical space. (c) Electrocoagulation of the uterine artery at its origin from the hypogastric artery.

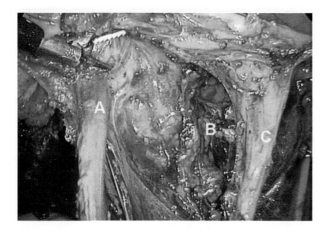

Figure 15.6 Unroofing of the right ureter (A) using harmonic shears. The paravesical space (B) and right obliterated umbilical artery (C) are identified.

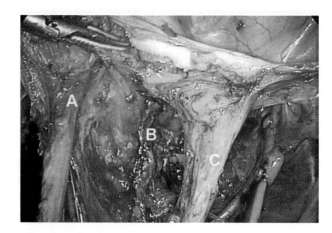

Figure 15.7 Resection of the right parametrium using harmonic shears. The ureter (A), paravesical space (B), and right obliterated umbilical artery (C) are revealed.

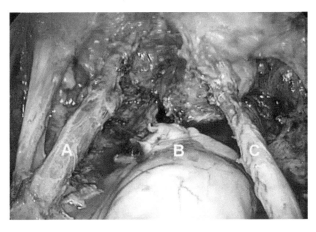

Figure 15.8 Panoramic view of the pelvis after removal of the specimen. Both ureters (A and C) have been dissected to the level of the bladder, and the rectosigmoid colon (B) can be seen in the center of the figure.

dense intestinal adhesions, a uterus larger than 14 cm, the presence of a large ventral hernia, pregnancy, and a body mass index greater than 35.

COMPLICATIONS AND THEIR PREVENTION

Complications can be divided into three groups: surgery-related, laparoscopy-related, and procedure-specific complications.

- Surgery-related complications are general surgical complications, such as pulmonary emboli, deep vein thrombosis, transfusion, fever, ileus, and small-bowel obstruction. We routinely use subcutaneous low-molecular-weight heparin or pneumatic compression devices until patients are fully ambulatory.

- Laparoscopy-related complications are conditions arising from the laparoscopy procedure, such as open conversion, incisional hernia, pneumomediastinum, and subcutaneous emphysema.
- Radical hysterectomy procedure-specific complications include ureteral injury, cystotomy, hydronephrosis, and ureterovaginal and vesicovaginal fistula.

SUGGESTED READING

- Piver MS, Rutledge F, Smith JP. Five classes of extended hysterectomy for women with cervical cancer. Obstet Gynecol 1974;44:265–72.
- Nezhat CR, Burrell MO, Nezhat FR, Benigno BB, Welander CE. Laparoscopic radical hysterectomy with paraaortic and pelvic node dissection. Am J Obstet Gynecol 1992;166:864–5.
- Nezhat CR, Nezhat FR, Burrell MO, et al. Laparoscopic radical hysterectomy and laparoscopically assisted vaginal radical hysterectomy with pelvic and paraaortic node dissection. J Gynecol Surg 1993;9:105–20.
- Zakashansky K, Chuang L, Gretz H, et al. A case-controlled study of total laparoscopic radical hysterectomy with pelvic lymphadenectomy versus radical abdominal hysterectomy in a fellowship training program. Int J Gynecol Cancer 2007; in press.
- Nezhat F, Mahdavi A, Nagarsheth NP. Total laparoscopic radical hysterectomy and pelvic lymphadenectomy using harmonic shears. J Minim Invasive Gynecol 2006;13:20–5.
- Nezhat F, Yadav J, Rahaman J, et al. Laparoscopic lymphadenectomy for gynecologic malignancies using ultrasonically activated shears: analysis of first 100 cases. Gynecol Oncol 2005;97:813–19.

16

Laparoscopic pelvic lymphadenectomy

Marie Plante and Michel Roy

The status of lymph nodes is the single most important prognostic marker in cervical cancer. In early-stage disease, the overall rate of pelvic lymph node metastasis is in the region of 15%. Traditionally, lymphadenectomy has always been performed through a midline incision. However, in the last two decades, advances in laparoscopic surgery have made it possible to perform a complete pelvic and para-aortic node dissection laparoscopically. The recent introduction of the sentinel node mapping technique has also allowed a better understanding of the lymphatic drainage of cervical cancers. It is now recognized that the most frequently involved lymph nodes in cancer of the cervix are those located medial to the external iliac vein and in the obturator fossa.

PROCEDURE

Operating room setup, port placement, and instrumentation

The procedure is performed under general anesthesia, with the patient in the supine position. Both arms are tucked alongside the body and a Foley catheter is placed in the bladder. The surgeon is placed on the right side of the patient to do left-sided lymph node dissection and the assistant is on the opposite side.

Laparoscopic pelvic lymphadenectomy is performed using a four-trocar technique. Two 10 mm trocars are placed in the subumbilical area and the suprapubic area, respectively, and 2– mm trocars are placed in the lateral flanks, almost midway between the anterior–superior iliac crest and the umbilicus

(Figure 16.1). After trocar placement, the patient is placed in a deep Tredelenburg position. A simple set of reusable instrumentation is required: a 5 mm tissue-grasper, 5 mm unipolar scissors, a 5 mm bipolar coagulation device, a 5 mm suction–irrigation device, and a 10 mm laparoscopic spoon to retrieve lymph nodes and to assist in retraction. Alternatively, lymph nodes can be collected into an Endopouch (Ethicon Endo-Surgery, Inc.) and retrieved via the suprapubic port. It is also prudent to have a clip-applicator device readily available in case of vascular injury.

Identification of the landmarks

Cancer of the cervix is known to spread preferentially via the lymphatic route. The lymphatic drainage follows the uterine artery pathway, exiting laterally at the level of the isthmus, traveling in the parametrial tissue, and then on to either the external iliac or obturator lymph node group. Occasionally, the lymphatic drainage bypasses the pelvic nodes and goes directly to the common iliac or para-aortic chain. The standard landmarks for node dissection are: the common iliac nodes proximally, the circumflex vein distally, the obturator nerve posteriorly, the pelvic sidewall laterally, and the superior vesical artery medially.

Opening of the retroperitoneal spaces

After trocar insertion, the upper abdomen and all the peritoneal surfaces are carefully inspected to exclude metastatic disease. Any suspicious areas, particularly in the posterior cul-de-sac, are biopsied and sent for frozen section. The lateral retroperitoneum is then

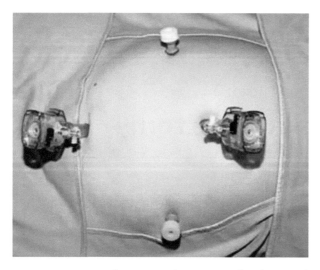

Figure 16.1 Trocar placement (the patient's head is on the right-hand side). The first 10 mm trocar is placed in the umbilicus and the other 10 mm trocar is placed suprapubically, two fingerbreaths above the pubic os. The lateral 5 mm trocars are placed midway between the anterosuperior iliac crest and the umbilicus.

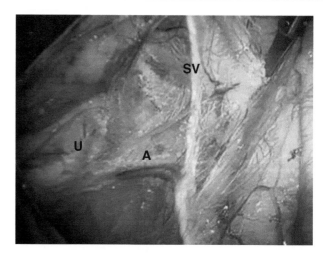

Figure 16.2 Opening of the retroperitoneal space (patient's right side). The broad ligament is retracted medially with the spoon thus retracting the ureter (U). The superior vesical artery (SV) and the uterine artery (A) are visualized.

opened with the unipolar scissors over the external iliac vessels, lateral to the infundibulopelvic (IP) ligament, and extended all the way down to the round ligament. After opening the retroperitoneal space further, the laparoscopic spoon is used to retract the broad ligament with the IP ligament and ureter medially. The obliterated umbilical artery or superior vesical artery is usually the first structure identified (Figure 16.2).

Obturator nodes

A space is then created just under the external iliac vein in its midportion and widened with the atraumatic grasper. This gives access to the lateral pelvic sidewall. All the node-bearing tissue between the sidewall and the superior vesical artery is grasped with the tissue-grasper and mobilized by blunt dissection and cauterized with the monopolar scissors as needed. As it is dissected free from its lateral and deep attachments, the obturator nerve is identified posteriorly. The nodal package should never be excised unless the obturator nerve has been identified with certainty. It is also important to remain anterior to the obturator nerve to avoid the complex vascular network located below the nerve, which can be a source of significant bleeding. The obturator lymph node package is mobilized cranially toward the bifurcation

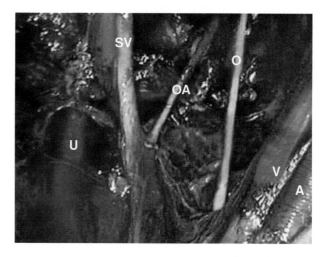

Figure 16.3 Obturator and external iliac area (patient's right side). The nodal package has been removed and all the retroperitoneal structures have completely skeletonized. Note the external iliac artery (A) and vein (V), the superior vesical artery (SV), the ureter (U), and the obturator nerve (O). An accessory obturator artery is also seen in this dissection (OA).

and dissected free; it is then removed with the spoon (Figure 16.3).

External iliac nodes

Next, the lymph nodes from the external iliac chain are removed. There are three groups of nodes in that area: (1) the lateral nodes situated between the external iliac artery and the psoas muscle; (2) the intermediate or interiliac nodes located between the external

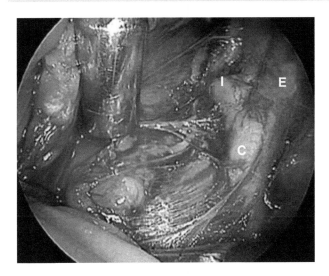

Figure 16.4 (a) Common iliac area (patient's right side). The nodal package has been removed. The common iliac artery (C) and the bifurcation leading to the division of the internal (I) and external (E) iliac arteries are well identified. The ureter has been retracted medially.

iliac artery and vein or anterior to the vein; and (3) the medial nodes, located between the external iliac vein and the obturator fossa. This last group of nodes is by far the most important lymph node chain to remove in cervical cancer.

Starting at the bifurcation and progressing caudally, the entire node-bearing tissue on the medial aspect of the iliac vein and between the iliac artery and vein is mobilized bluntly with the scissors and atraumatic grasper, and then removed. The external iliac artery and vein are completely skeletonized (Figure 16.3). Technically, the lateral node chain between the external iliac artery and the psoas muscle should be removed all the way down to the circumflex vein. However, with our current knowledge of the lymphatic drainage of the cervix, it appears that these lymph nodes are very rarely involved in cervical cancer. Their removal is actually responsible for a significant part of the morbidity associated with the lymphadenectomy, namely injury to the femorocutaneous nerve, bleeding, and peripheral lymphedema. Therefore, a less extensive dissection of the lateral nodal chain is recommended.

Bifurcation and common iliac nodes

Once the external iliac nodal tissue has been removed, it is usually easy to locate the bifurcation of the iliac artery. Residual nodal tissue can be removed cautiously in that area. Next, the common iliac artery is delineated. It is extremely important at this point to locate the ureter, as it crosses the common iliac artery approximately 1 cm above the bifurcation. Once identified, the ureter is mobilized medially with the spoon along with the medial sheath of the broad ligament and the IP ligament. Nodal tissue overlying the first 2 cm of the common iliac artery is removed (Figure 16.4).

COMPLICATIONS

Complications secondary to lymphadenectomy include trauma to the retroperitoneal vascular structures, damage to the obturator nerve and femorocutaneous nerve (paresthesia of the upper thigh), lymphocele formation (usually asymptomatic), and lymphedema (rare in the absence of adjuvant radiation therapy). The conversion rate to laparotomy is low, particularly with increasing experience. Large published series indicate that the complication rate of laparoscopic pelvic lymphadenectomy is actually quite low and compares favourably with the abdominal approach.

SUGGESTED READING

- Querleu D, Leblanc E, Cartron G, et al. Audit of preoperative and early complications of laparoscopic lymph node dissection in 1000 gynecologic cancer patients. Am J Obstet Gynecol 2006;195:1287–92.
- Kohler C, Klemm P, Schau A, et al. Introduction of transperitoneal lymphadenectomy in a gynecologic oncology center: analysis of 650 laparoscopic pelvic and/or paraaortic transperitoneal lymphadenectomies. Gynecol Oncol 2004;95:52–61.
- Kehoe SM, Abu-Rustum N. Transperitoneal laparoscopic pelvic and paraaortic lymphadenectomy in gynecologic cancers. Curr Treat Options Oncol 2006;7:93–101.

17

Laparoscopic treatment of urinary incontinence

Rose C Kung

The two most common surgical procedures that provide higher long-term success rates in the treatment of urinary incontinence are retropubic suspensions (i.e., Burch) and slings. Burch procedures rely on elevation of the bladder neck using sutures to suspend the paravaginal fascia to Cooper's ligaments. This requires that the vaginal length be adequate and that there be mobility of the bladder neck. Typically, Burch suspensions are performed as primary procedures. Sling procedures are reserved for cases with recurrent stress incontinence or cases considered as high risks for failure from a Burch suspension. These include decreased bladder neck mobility secondary to extensive scarring, intrinsic urethral sphincter deficiency with the typical drainpipe urethra, as well as individuals with chronic bronchitis, asthma, chronic steroid use, congenital tissue weakness, severe obesity, or constipation, smokers, and those participating in recreational and/or occupational activities that include heavy lifting or high impact exposure.

The purpose of the sling procedure is to restore the support of the urethrovesical junction by compressing the proximal urethra during episodes of increases in intraabdominal pressure. Sling procedures may be performed transvaginally (i.e., TVT), transabdominally, or laparoscopically using a two-team approach. The success rate of a laparoscopic approach to a sling procedure is 88.6% and the complication rate is 27%.

PROCEDURE

Laparoscopic Burch suspension

Extraperitoneal approach

Ideal patients for an extraperitoneal approach are those who have not had an abdominal incision, particularly a midline incision.

- A disposable balloon device is first inserted anterior to the posterior rectus sheath through a small infraumbilical incision. The balloon is distended with water or air using a bulbar syringe to dissect the anterior peritoneum from the overlying rectus muscle. This is usually done under direct vision. In those with previous midline operation scar, scarring will cause the balloon to dissect on one side of the retropubic space and potentially rupture the underlying peritoneum and/or the balloon.
- Once the space of Retzius is created, the balloon is removed and replaced with a Hasson trocar and carbon dioxide (CO_2) is insufflated. Two 10–12 mm lateral ports are inserted lateral to the inferior epigastric vessels for suturing. Often the amount of space is no more than 500 cm^3 volume, and careful placement of the lateral ports is crucial to avoid puncturing the peritoneum as well as injuring inferior epigastric vessels. Prophylactic cauterization of vessels commonly found superior to Cooper's ligaments are recommended.

Dissection is carried out laterally to the aberrant obturator vessels that cross Cooper's ligaments (Figure 17.1).

- We use nonabsorbable sutures such as Prolene or Gore-Tex. Either one or two sutures may be placed at the level of the bladder neck as defined with the aid of a vaginal finger placed just inferior to the 20–30 cm³ Foley balloon. Dissection of the bladder from lateral to medial to visualize the paravaginal fascia usually avoids unnecessary trauma to the detrusor and excessive bleeding. Prophylactic use of bipolar cautery of vessels over the paravaginal fascia will minimize blood loss. Full-thickness figure-of-eight bites through the paravaginal fascia will also minimize blood loss.
- If two sutures are used on each side, the inferior suture is introduced from the contralateral port and the superior suture from the ipsilateral port to avoid suture entanglement. For example, if one is suturing on the right paravaginal fascia and Cooper's ligaments, the first suture should be introduced from the left trocar and the second suture (more proximal) from the right trocar. Both sutures from the same side are tied after penetration of Cooper's ligaments using extracorporeal knot-tying techniques. Excessive elevation of the vaginal tissues should be avoided due to potential complications of urinary retention, voiding dysfunction, and ureteral obstruction (Figure 17.2).

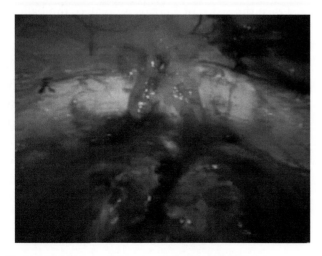

Figure 17.1 Space of Retzius with Cooper's ligaments.

- Cystoscopy is recommended to rule out inadvertent suture placement through the bladder mucosa and ureteral obstruction. Indigo carmine is usually given intravenously a few minutes prior to cystoscopy, or methylene blue may be used 20–30 minutes prior to cystoscopy. Intravenous furosemide 10 mg may also be given to reduce time interval between intravenous indigo carmine injection and visualization of the dye cystoscopically. Suprapubic or urethral catheters can be used (Figure 17.3). Patients are taught to perform intermittent self-catheterization either preoperatively or postoperatively as needed.

Intraperitoneal approach.

- Entry into the space of Retzius can be achieved using monopolar scissors, harmonic scalpel or CO_2 laser. Initially, the bladder may be filled with 150–200 cm³ of water through the Foley catheter to facilitate visualization of the outline of the bladder abdominally. The pubic tubercle is identified in the midline. Usually the peritoneal incision starts 6 cm above the symphysis in the midline and is carried out laterally just medial to the obliterated umbilical vessels. The incision is curved slightly inferiorly as one approaches laterally so that the peritoneal flap will independently remain deflected inferiorly without the need for traction. The incision should be sufficiently deep to encounter the loose areolar tissue beneath the rectus muscle, leaving the majority of the fatty tissue attached to the peritoneal reflection posteriorly.
- Often one encounters small vessels running parallel to Cooper's ligaments that can be cauterized prophylactically with bipolar cautery. This avoids bleeding from a suture going through Cooper's ligaments that could injure the vessel. After the Burch sutures are tied and cystoscopy is completed, the peritoneum is closed either with a running absorbable suture or with staples. This avoids potential bowel herniation into the space of Retzius. The advantages of an intraperitoneal approach include full visualization and inspection of both upper and lower abdomen and pelvis as well as plication of uterosacral ligaments, culdoplasty, or a Moschcowitz suture to obliterate the cul-de-sac if desired.

(a)

(b)

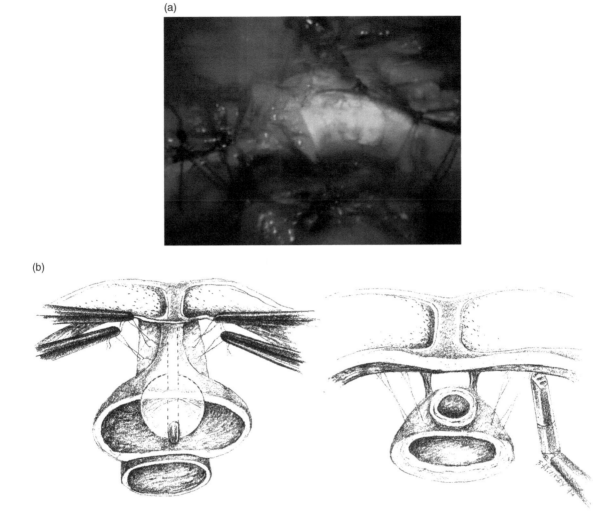

Figure 17.2 (a) Placement of Burch sutures (a total of 4) along the paravaginal fascia tied to Cooper's ligaments, showing suture bridges. (b) Diagrammatic representation.

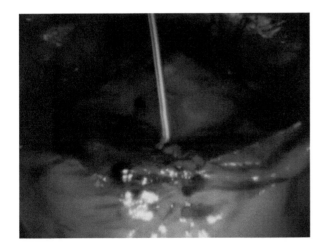

Figure 17.3 Insertion of the suprapubic catheter under direct visualization both laparoscopically and cystoscopically.

Laparoscopic slings

- Access to the retropubic space for a laparoscopic sling procedure is initially similar to that for the laparoscopic Burch suspension. In cases where a retropubic suspension has previously failed, excessive, dense scarring in the retropubic space can be problematic and the risk of cystotomy is increased. Filling the bladder partially with 100–200 cm^3 of methylene blue in normal saline can aid in dissection and early recognition of injury. Careful, meticulous dissection using a CO_2 laser is extremely useful, and approaching from a lateral to medial direction (from normal tissue to scarred tissue) is easier.

- Vaginally, the bladder is sharply dissected from the anterior vaginal wall through a vertical midline incision, freeing up any adhesions. An imbricating suture of 2-0 chromic or 2-0 Biosyn is used to support the bladder neck. Periurethral tunnels are created using sharp dissection and a 1.5–2.0 cm-wide piece of Prolene mesh is introduced through these tunnels using long dressing forceps. The perineal membrane on either side is perforated under laparoscopic guidance and the arms of the mesh are gently retrieved with blunt graspers. Once the mesh is introduced into the retropubic space, the pneumoperitoneum will be reduced suddenly. By using a wet sponge to plug up the periurethral tunnel vaginally, the second arm of the mesh can then be introduced vaginally on the opposite side while maintaining adequate visualization laparoscopically.

- The mesh is secured vaginally to the bladder neck using 2-0 chromic or 2-0 Polysorb sutures to prevent the mesh from rolling higher up on the bladder. Laparoscopically, the mesh is sutured to Cooper's ligament without tension using 0 Prolene sutures (Figure 17.4). Methylene blue dye is introduced into the bladder via a Foley catheter to ensure that the bladder mucosa is intact. Occasionally, bleeding will occur from the periurethral tunnels. This can be controlled by inserting two small pieces of Surgicel – one in each tunnel – which also helps maintain the

pneumoperitoneum and allow the laparoscopic surgeons to continue with their suturing of the mesh. The vaginal incision is closed with running 2-0 Polysorb suture. Closure of peritoneum is done with a 2-0 Maxon suture if an intraperitoneal approach is utilized. The CO_2 is released and the fascia closed with 1 Polysorb.

- Foley catheters are removed on the first postoperative day and residuals are done only if patients are symptomatic or unable to void after 6 hours. The Foley catheter is left in until the next morning if the residual is > 300 cm^3.

COMPLICATIONS AND THEIR PREVENTION

- Potential intraoperative complications include bleeding, as well as bladder, bowel, and ureteric injuries. These are more common in cases with previous abdominal/pelvic procedures.

- Inadvertent cystotomies are repaired laparoscopically using 2-0 or 3-0 Polysorb or Vicryl sutures in either a single or a double layer in a running fashion, depending upon the size of the defect. Filling the bladder with methylene blue via a Foley catheter will determine whether small defects still exist and need to be repaired. Usually, leaving the catheter in place for 5–7 days and antibiotic treatment will allow adequate healing. A cystogram can be done prior to removal of the Foley catheter to ensure that there is no leak.

- Ureteric injuries from sutures placed too laterally during a Burch suspension can be detected via intraoperative cystoscopic examination. The sutures can be cut and replaced.

- Inadvertent enterotomy can also be repaired laparoscopically in two layers; however, it is recommended that a General Surgery consult be obtained.

- Postoperative complications include cystitis, wound infection, mesh erosion, urinary retention, and overactive bladder. Treatment of cystitis involves short course of antibiotic therapy, usually Macrobid (nitrofurantoin) or Septra DS (trimethoprim–sulfamethoxazole, double strength). This can occur despite antibiotic prophylaxis with 1 g of Ancef IV (cefazolin) preoperatively.

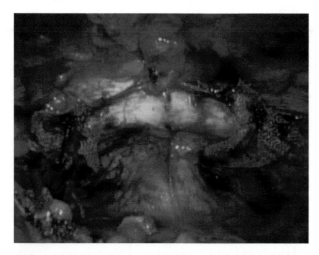

Figure 17.4 Attachment of the polypropylene mesh to Cooper's ligaments without tension in the laparoscopic sling procedure.

- Urinary retention, which can occur in 10–15% of cases, can be dealt with by an indwelling Foley catheter, to be removed every 3–4 days until residuals are <100 cm^3. To minimize the risk of urinary retention and voiding dysfunction, one should avoid applying excessive tension on the sling. The arms of the sling should lie flat without tension when anchored to Cooper's ligament.
- Postoperative de novo bladder instability may occur up to 10% of cases, but is usually self-limiting, lasting up to 3 months. Rarely are anticholinergic agents required on a long-term basis.
- Mesh erosion can occur in individuals with atrophic vaginal tissues. This can be avoided in most cases by prescribing local estrogen therapy for a few months prior to the surgery (i.e., Premarin vaginal cream, Vagifem, or Estring), making a full-thickness incision in the vagina, repairing the vaginal incision without excessive tension, and using local estrogen therapy postoperatively.
- Vaginal packing is suggested if a posterior repair is done concomitantly to avoid midline vaginal adhesions from the anterior to the posterior wall.

The patient is instructed to avoid intercourse for at least 6–8 weeks. If, after a few months, the mesh is still exposed, this can usually be trimmed in the office, although rarely the patient requires removal of the mesh in the operating room.

SUGGESTED READING

- Horbach NS. Suburethral sling procedures. In: Ostergard DR, Bent AE, eds. Urogynecology and Urodynamics: Theory and Practice, 4th edn. Baltimore: Williams & Wilkins, 1996:569–79.
- Vancaillie TG, Schuessler W. Laparoscopic bladder neck suspension. J Laparoendosc Surg 1991;1: 169–73.
- Liu CY, Paek WS. Laparoscopic retropubic colposuspension. J Am Assoc Gynecol Laparosc 1993;1: 31–5.
- Hofenfellner R, Petrie E. Sling procedures in surgery. In: Stanton SL, Tanagho E, eds. Surgery of Female Incontinence, 2nd edn. Berlin: Springer-Verlag, 1986:105–13.
- Von Theobald P, Lucas J, Barjot P, et al. Feasibility of the laparoscopic sub-urethral sling procedure. J Gynecol Obstet Biol Reprod 1999;28:529–33.

18A

Laparoscopic appendectomy

Bulent Berker, Jaime Ocampo, Mario Nutis, and Camran Nezhat

To date, there have been more than two dozen prospective randomized trials showing that laparoscopic appendectomy produces better outcomes for patients with suspected acute appendicitis than conventional open appendectomy. Appendectomy is advisable after other laparoscopic procedures have been completed.

PROCEDURE

Incidental appendectomy

- After the pelvis is inspected, the appendix is identified, mobilized, and examined. Periappendiceal or pericecal adhesions are lysed. The meso-appendix is coagulated with bipolar forceps or clipped and cut to skeletonize the appendix (Figures 18A.1–18A.3). Fecal contents are milked toward the tip of the appendix by using a grasper over an area 2 cm from the cecum. Two Endoloop sutures (Ethicon Endo-Surgery, Inc.) are passed sequentially through one of the 5 mm suprapubic trocar sleeves and looped around the base of the appendix next to each other (Figure 18A.4). A third Endoloop suture is applied 5 mm distal to the first two sutures. Hulka clips (used for tubal sterilization) can be used also to secure the proximal and distal portions of the appendix. The appendix is cut between the two sets of sutures, using laser or laparoscopic scissors (Figure 18A.5). The luminal portion of the appendiceal stump is seared with the CO_2 laser, providone–iodine (Betadine) solution

may be applied, and the tissues are irrigated copiously with lactated Ringer's solution. A pursestring or Z-suture can be placed in the cecum to bury the appendiceal stump, although there appears to be no advantage to its invagination. Simple ligation simplifies the technical procedure and shortens the operating time.

- An Endoloop suture can be placed around the distal tip of the appendix as a substitute for a grasping instrument during initial mobilization and excision of the appendix. Once the appendix is free, the suture is used to pull the appendix into a 5 or 10 mm accessory trocar sleeve. The trocar sleeve is removed from the suprapubic incision with the appendix contained within it. Alternatively, the appendix can be placed inside an endoscopic pouch, minimizing contact between contaminated tissue and the pelvis.

- Stapling devices make laparoscopic appendectomy easier and faster. The multifire stapler is introduced through a 12 mm suprapubic midline incision and applied directly across the entire mesoappendix and appendix. In a single motion, the entire appendix and its meso-appendix are clipped and cut (Figure 18A.6). The stapler's operation should not be hindered by contact with surrounding tissue, and the cecum must be free from attachments. In addition, appendiceal contents do not leak intraperitoneally, and the larger trocar sleeve allows easier removal of the separated appendix. The disadvantages to the stapling device are its cost and the need to use a 12 mm trocar.

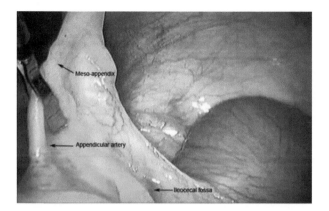

Figure 18A.1 The meso-appendix is coagulated with bipolar forceps.

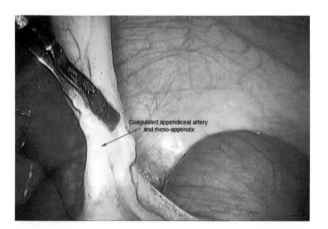

Figure 18A.2 Coagulated meso-appendix and appendiceal artery.

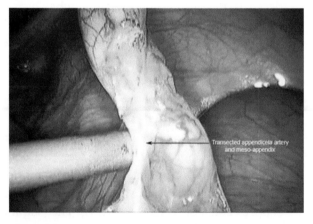

Figure 18A.3 The base of the meso-appendix can be cut with the CO_2 laser.

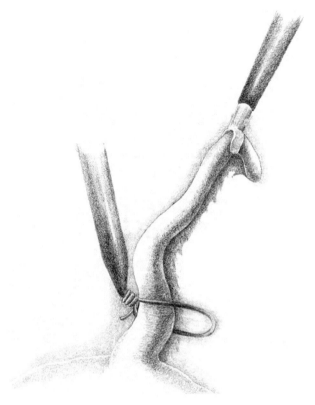

Figure 18A.4 Placement of a pretied ligature (Endoloop).

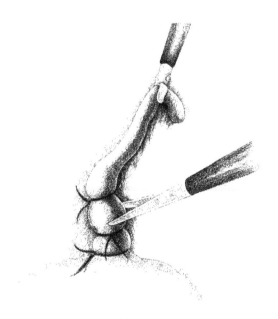

Figure 18A.5 Transection of the appendix between the second and third ligatures.

Laparoscopic appendectomy for appendicitis

- The procedure is similar to an incidental appendectomy, except that the appendix is edematous and possibly more fragile. In removing the appendix at its base, a sufficient stump is left to prevent spillage of luminal contents from the pedicle. An alternative procedure is to place Hulka clips on the base of the inflamed appendix and then control the blood supply in the meso-appendix with electrocoagulation, hemaclips, or a multifire

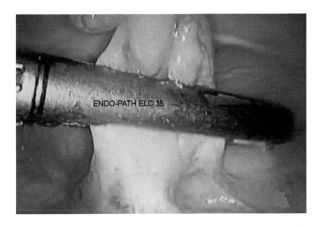

Figure 18A.6 The multifire stapler is inserted through a 12 mm trocar sleeve and applied directly across the meso-appendix and appendix. In a single motion, the entire appendix and the meso-appendix are clipped and cut.

stapling device. If an inflamed appendix is removed laparoscopically, a larger trocar may be needed to ease its removal, and the operative site is irrigated copiously.

Laparoscopic appendectomy for perforated appendicitis and appendiceal abscess

The safety and efficacy of laparoscopic appendectomy for perforated and gangrenous appendicitis remains to be established in randomized controlled trials.

COMPLICATIONS AND THEIR PREVENTION

- A significant difference was found in the incidence of postoperative small-bowel obstruction when invagination was compared with stump ligation. In the invagination group, there were six instances of bowel obstruction (1.6%), while the stump ligation group included only one patient who became obstructed postoperatively (0.3%). This difference in complications may be related to the high incidence of adhesions found in more than 70% of patients with pursestring or Z-suture placement.
- Complications include stump blowout, wound infection, hemorrhage, and postoperative ileus.

SUGGESTED READING

- Kumar R, Erian M, Sinnot S, Knoesen R, Kimble R. Laparoscopic appendectomy in modern gynecology. J Am Assoc Gynecol Laparosc 2002;9:252–63.
- Reiertsen O, Larsen S, Trondsen E, et al. Randomized controlled trial with sequential design of laparoscopic versus conventional appendicectomy. Br J Surg 1997;84:842–7.
- Cervini P, Smith LC, Urbach DR. The surgeon on call is a strong factor determining the use of a laparoscopic approach for appendectomy. Surg Endosc 2002; 16:1774–7.
- Harris RS, Foster WG, Surrey MW, et al. Appendiceal disease in women with endometriosis and right lower quadrant pain. J Am Assoc Gynecol Laparosc 2001; 8:536–41.
- Berker B, Lashay N, Davarpanah R, Marziali M, Nezhat CH, Nezhat C. Laparoscopic appendectomy in patients with endometriosis. J Minim Invasive Gynecol 2005; 12:206–9.

18B

Laparoscopic bowel resection

Andrew A Shelton, Camran Nezhat, Ceana Nezhat, and Farr Nezhat

Endometrial implants involving the distal ileum frequently require mobilization of the distal ileum and right colon to facilitate a laparoscopically assisted ileocolic resection with an ileo–ascending colostomy or a laparoscopically assisted ileal resection with an ileo–ileostomy. (Figure 18B.1–18B.4).

PROCEDURE

Ileocolic resection and small-bowel resection

Preoperative preparation includes a mechanical bowel preparation using polyethylene glycol (Golytely) or sodium phosphate (Fleet Phosphosoda). Antibiotics covering gram-negative rods and anaerobes are given within 60 minutes of the incision.

- The patient is placed in a steep Trendelenburg position with the left side down to facilitate mobilization of the small bowel out of the pelvis. The first assistant, standing on the patient's left side, retracts the small bowel out of the pelvis, exposing the posterior attachment of the distal ileal mesentery in the patient's right lower quadrant. The surgeon, standing between the patient's legs or on the patient's right side, then grasps the cecum or appendix, retracting it toward the patient's head, exposing the retroperitoneal attachments and placing them on tension.
- The peritoneum of the ileal mesentery is divided with electrocautery from the third portion of the duodenum to the cecum. The ileal and right colon

mesentery can be mobilized free from the retroperitoneum using blunt and sharp dissection, exposing the right ovarian vessels, the right ureter, the second and third portions of the duodenum, and the right kidney. The colon is mobilized up the level of the hepatic flexure. Leaving the lateral attachments of the ascending colon intact to this point facilitates placing traction on the right colon. After completing the posterior mobilization of the colon, the lateral peritoneal attachment of the right colon is easily divided with electrocautery, with medial retraction of the colon. If necessary, the attachment of the hepatic flexure and the right side of the gastrocolic ligament can be divided with the LigaSure, completely mobilizing the right colon.

- After fully mobilizing the colon and ileal mesentery, the bowel is ready to be resected. This can be accomplished entirely intracorporeally using the LigaSure for mesenteric division, and the Endo GIA stapler (US Surgical) for division of the bowel and creation of a stapled side-to-side functional end-to-end anastomosis. For retraction of the specimen, we favor enlarging the midline or right lower quadrant incision, extraction of the segment of bowel to be resected, and an extracorporeal anastomosis. After fully mobilizing the colon and distal small-bowel mesenteries, the right colon and terminal ileum are easily prolapsed out through a small 4–5 cm incision in the right lower quadrant or midline. The bowel proximal and distal or the endometrial implant is divided with a GIA stapler. The mesentery is

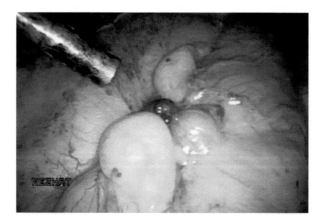

Figure 18B.1 Constrictive lesion of the sigmoid colon.

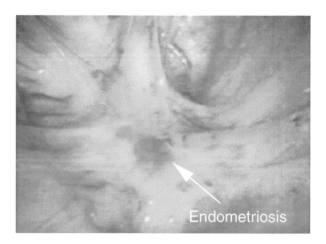

Figure 18B.3 Superficial endometriosis of the rectum.

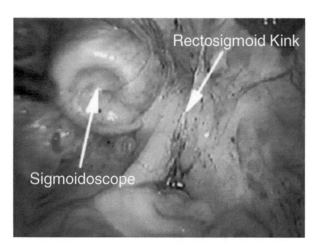

Figure 18B.2 Infiltrative endometriosis of the rectosigmoid.

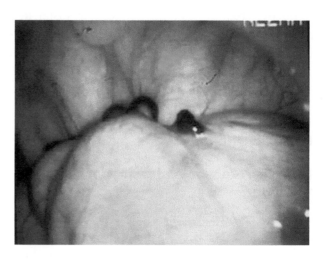

Figure 18B.4 Multiple endometriosis on the sipmoid colon.

divided with the LigaSure, and the specimen is removed.

- The antimesenteric corners of the staple lines are then divided, and a side-to-side anastomosis is created with a third firing of the GIA stapler. The remaining enterotomy can then be sutured closed or stapled closed with another firing of the GIA stapler, or a TA stapler, and the bowel placed back intraperitoneally.

Segmental colon resection

The most common segment of colon requiring resection is the sigmoid. The first assistant, standing on the patient's left side, first grasps the sigmoid colon or its mesentery using a traumatic graspers (e.g., an endo-Babcock), and retracts the sigmoid colon in a ventral fashion toward the patient's abdominal wall, placing traction on the medial portion of the sigmoid mesentery.

- Using electrocautery, the peritoneum of the sigmoid mesentery is separated from the sacral promontory to the take-off of the left colic artery. Using blunt and sharp dissection, the sigmoid mesentery is mobilized off of the retroperitoneum, exposing the gonadal vessels and the left ureter.
- The superior rectal artery can be isolated and divided with a device such as the LigaSure or an Endo GIA stapler with a vascular cartridge. The descending colon can then be bluntly mobilized

free from the retroperitoneum. Leaving the lateral attachments of the sigmoid and descending colon intact to this point preserves the ability to provide traction to the otherwise-mobile colon and facilitates dissection. The colon can then be retracted medially and the lateral peritoneal attachments divided as far proximally as necessary. If necessary, the splenic flexure can be mobilized laparoscopically.

- The mesentery at the level of the rectosigmoid junction can then be divided with the LigaSure, and the rectosigmoid junction can be divided with an endoscopic GIA-type stapler passed through the right lower quadrant port site.

- If the patient is undergoing a concomitant laparoscopic hysterectomy, the vaginal cuff can be left open and the proximal end delivered out through the vagina. The mesentery of the colon proximal to the endometrioma and the colon are divided, and the specimen can be passed from the field.

- The anvil of a circular stapler is placed in the open end of the descending colon and secured in place with a pursestring suture, and the colon is retracted back intraperitoneally.

- If a hysterectomy is not being performed, the left lower quadrant port is removed and the incision enlarged 4–5 cm, and the colon is removed and similarly resected. The head of the stapler is then passed transanally by the assistant and opened through the apex of the stapled-off rectum. Laparoscopic anvil graspers are useful in facilitating connection of the anvil and the stapler, which is then closed and fired, creating a double-stapled colorectal anastomosis.

Anterior disc excision

Deeper lesions on the anterior rectal wall require more extensive resection, but a formal low anterior resection is not necessarily required.

- A full-thickness excision of the anterior rectal wall can be performed using electrocautery or carbon dioxide laser after laparoscopic mobilization of the rectum. The resulting proctotomy is then closed transversely with an Endo GIA stapler, or sutures are placed laparoscopically.

- The use of a circular stapler is useful for anterior rectal endometriomas that occupy less than one-third of the circumference of the rectal wall and are < 2 cm in size. The rectum is laparoscopically mobilized anteriorly and laterally, encompassing the endometriosis lesion on the anterior rectal wall. Sufficient mobilization of the vagina off the rectal wall is performed down to normal, healthy, soft, supple rectum. The circular stapler is inserted transanally, with the anvil in place. It is then opened, with the area to be excised placed in the hollow between the anvil and the shoulder of the stapler. A suture or tie held by graspers on either side of the rectum is then used to place downward pressure on the portion of the rectum to be excised, while upward pressure is then placed on the stapler. This places the area to be excised within the stapler. The stapler is then closed and fired, excising a portion of the anterior rectal wall without narrowing the lumen of the rectum. The specimen should be examined to confirm excision of the nodule with a margin of normal rectum.

- Larger lesions can be treated in a similar fashion if they are partially transected, leaving a portion on the posterior vaginal or uterine wall and only 2 cm on the anterior rectal wall. Woods, Heriot, and Chen reported results using this technique on 30 patients. Although they found morbidity in 13% of cases, only one had an anastomotic leak. Other complications included difficulty with stapler extraction, minor bleeding from the staple line requiring no further treatment, and a patient who presented with pelvic pain and fevers, but no radiographic evidence of an anastomotic leak. The advantages of this technique are absence of leakage of intestinal content into the abdominal cavity, and no need for suturing deep in the pelvis. Similar success using this technique has been reported by others, with no anastomotic leaks.

Anterior resection and low anterior resection

An anterior resection is defined as an anastomosis between the colon and the intraperitoneal rectum, while a low anterior resection implies an anastomosis between the colon and the extraperitoneal rectum.

- The operation proceeds similarly to that described for segmental resection of the sigmoid colon.

However, rather than stapling the rectosigmoid junction, the rectum is mobilized below the level of the endometriosis. The blood supply of the rectum travels within the mesorectum, entering the mesorectum proximally as the superior rectal artery or inferiorly from the pelvic floor as the inferior rectal artery.

- The mesorectum is contained within a layer of fascia known as the fascia propria. Therefore, after incising the lateral and anterior peritoneal attachment of the rectum, if one is in the correct plane, it is possible to mobilize the rectum posteriorly, laterally, and anteriorly to the level of the levator ani muscles in an avascular plane, with appropriate traction and counter-traction on the rectum.

- Once the rectum is sufficiently mobilized below the involved segment, the mesorectum must be divided with a device such as the LigaSure and the rectum transected with a stapling device. The bowel is resected, and the anastomosis is created and checked as described in the section on sigmoid resection.

COMPLICATIONS AND THEIR PREVENTION

- Following segmental colon resection, both proximal and distal rings should be inspected to insure that they are intact. Inflating the rectum through a rigid proctoscope under water with the proximal bowel occluded represents a 'leak-test'. Any air leak can then be reinforced with laparoscopically placed sutures. Care should be taken to adhere to sound surgical principles, including creation of a well-vascularized, tension-free anastomosis to minimize the risk of anastomotic leak.

- Minor bleeding from the staple line requires no further treatment.

SUGGESTED READING

- A comparison of laparoscopically assisted and open colectomy for colon cancer. N Engl J Med 2004; 350:2050–9.
- Lacy AM, Garcia-Valdecasas JC, Delgado S, et al. Laparoscopy-assisted colectomy versus open colectomy for treatment of non-metastatic colon cancer: a randomized trial. Lancet 2002;359:2224–9.
- Milsom JW, Hammerhofer KA, Bohm B, et al. Prospective, randomized trial comparing laparoscopic vs. conventional surgery for refractory ileocolic Crohn's disease. Dis Colon Rectum 2001;44:1–8; discussion 8–9.
- Marcello PW, Milsom JW, Wong SK, et al. Laparoscopic restorative proctocolectomy: case-matched comparative study with open restorative proctocolectomy. Dis Colon Rectum 2000;43:604–8.
- Woods RJ, Heriot AG, Chen FC. Anterior rectal wall excision for endometriosis using the circular stapler. Aust NZ J Surg 2003;73:647–8.
- Jatan AK, Solomon MJ, Young J, Cooper M, Pathma-Nathan N. Laparoscopic management of rectal endometriosis. Dis Colon Rectum 2006;49:169–74.

19

Laparoscopic pelvic floor repair

Thomas L Lyons

ANTERIOR WALL – THE LATERAL DEFECTS

Most urogynecologists would agree that, with anterior wall mobility, a Burch retropubic colposuspension (see Chapter 17) or a suburethral sling procedure such as a tension-free vaginal tape (TVT) or a transobturator tape (TOT) procedure is the treatment of choice for urinary stress incontinence. If the patient has other defects, including cystocele, enterocele, or rectocele, a different approach is necessary.

Cystocele results from separation of the vaginal endopelvic fascia from its natural attachment to the arcus tendineous or the White's line of the pelvis (Figures 19.1 and 19.2). Although rare, a midline defect in this fascial unit results in a midline cystocele. Cystocele can be accompanied by anterior enterocele. Lateral separation of the fascia is more common. It causes unilateral or bilateral paravaginal defects. These are best treated using site-specific repair with restoration of the fascial attachments. Complete repair of all defects gives long-term clinical success.

Figures 19.1–19.3 show anatomic defects that require treatment. Figure 19.4 demonstrates a laparoscopic view of defects in the retropubic space.

Procedure

1. The space of Retzius is entered using either a preperitoneal or a transperitoneal approach. With the preperitoneal approach, we recommend an open laparoscopy technique with entry down to the posterior sheath of the rectus fascia (Figure 19.5).
2. The trocar is then anchored after gentle blunt dissection of this space. The pneumoperitoneum is allowed to complete the dissection of the space. The laparoscope itself can be used as a blunt dissector. Alternatively, a balloon cannula or an optically guided trocar can be used to facilitate the dissection.
3. Most patients with paravaginal defects also have posterior wall defects that have to be repaired first. Similarly, other procedures, including hysterectomy, have to be completed first.
4. An incision is made 2.5 cm above the symphysis pubis (identified by palpation) and the bladder is filled with saline temporarily until the space is identified. The incision is extended laterally to the obliterated umbilical ligaments and slightly caudad toward the symphysis. Blunt dissection brings the operator into the space. Anatomic

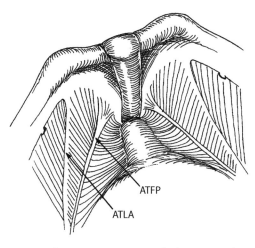

Figure 19.1 Schematic anatomy of the retropubic space. ATLC = Arcus tendineus levatoris ani. ATFP = archus tendineus fasciae pelvis.

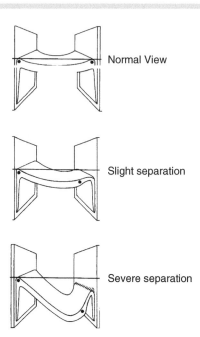

Figure 19.3 Laparoscopic anatomy of the retropubic space. IS = ischial spine.

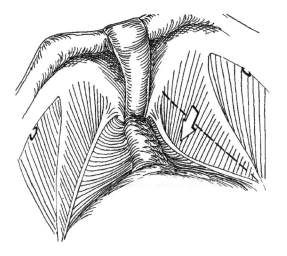

Figure 19.2 Schematic anatomy of paravaginal defect (see arrow).

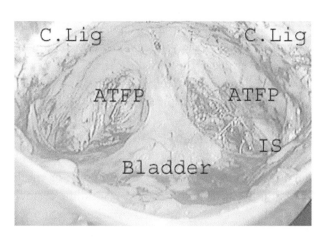

Figure 19.4 Laparoscopic view of retropubic space and paravaginal defects.

landmarks are the symphysis pubis, Cooper's ligaments, obturator canal and neurovascular bundle, ischial spines, arcus tendineous, vaginal endopelvic fascia, bladder, and urethra.

5. Removal of fat or areolar tissue allows identification of the paravaginal defect. This defect

is closed using interrupted sutures or a variation of a running stitch with nonabsorbable sutures. The initial suture should be placed close to the ischial spine on the lateral wall. This is the deepest point in the pelvis, and will be the first obscured if any bleeding occurs during

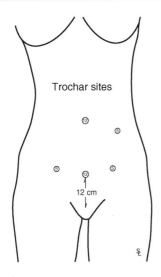

Figure 19.5 Trochar sites.

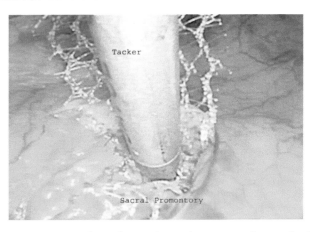

Figure 19.8 Tracking the mesh to the anterior longitudinal ligament over the sacral promontory.

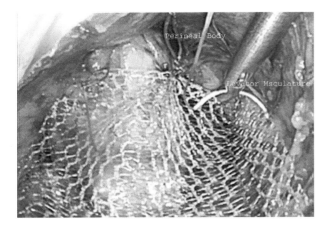

Figure 19.6 Rectovaginal space. Mesh being applied to levator fascia.

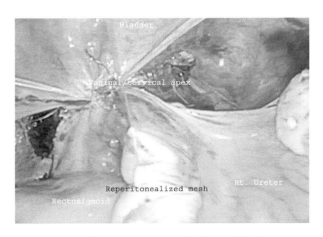

Figure 19.9 Mesh is retroperitonealized completely.

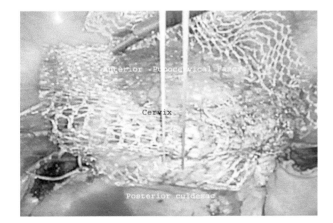

Figure 19.7 Y-mesh applied to anterior and posterior vaginal fascia.

the suturing process. The vaginal endopelvic fascia is reattached to the arcus until the defect is closed.

6. After bilateral repair of the paravaginal defect, the Burch procedure is performed by placing two similar sutures on each side 1–2 cm lateral to the urethra (Chapter 17). We use figure-of-eight sutures into the endopelvic fascia and then through the Cooper's ligament, further stabilizing the anterior wall and correcting the anterolateral wall defects. These sutures are placed first at the midurethral site and then at the urethra–vesicle (UV) junction. Burch sutures should not

be placed above this UV junction lest a funneling effect be caused, creating greater tendency for urinary stress incontinence.

7. After completion of the 'paravaginal plus' procedure in the laparoscopic approach, the operator can inspect the vaginal vault. The increased intraabdominal pressure due to the pneumoperitoneum allows the surgeon to evaluate the success of the repair.

8. A cystoscopy is then performed to evaluate urethral patency and to ascertain absence of suture material in the bladder.

9. The anterior wall peritoneum is closed with a pursestring suture using 2-0 polyglycolic acid.

10. Bladder drainage is facilitated with a Foley catheter, which is removed in the recovery room. The patient is allowed to void 5 hours later; if unsuccessful, the catheter is left in situ overnight. More than 90% of patients will void spontaneously on the day of surgery, and less than 1% of patients require self-catheterization.

11. Patients are required to observe pelvic rest for 6–8 weeks postoperatively.

THE POSTERIOR WALL

In contrast to anterior wall defects, those of the posterior wall are less understood. Although a posterior arcus tendineous has been identified in magnetic resonance imaging (MRI) studies of nulliparous patients, it has not been seen in cadavers or at surgical dissection. Due to the lack of long-term success in treating posterior wall relaxation, most surgeons use grafting material – mostly meshes.

Procedure

1. The mesh can be placed as part of a posterior wall/enterocele repair laparoscopically by simply dissecting the rectovaginal space and attaching the mesh with permanent sutures. The mesh is inserted via a 10 mm trocar. This procedure, combined with a McCall's culdoplasty and vault

suspension, creates a sturdy wall that is unlikely to fail.

2. Better than vault suspension is sacral colpopexy or sacral colpoperineopexy. We prefer the latter. Here, a Y-shaped graft is fashioned with one arm placed on the posterior wall and the short arm wrapped over the cervix or vault apex and attached to the anterior pubocervical fascia (Figures 19.6 and 19.7).

3. The remaining arm of the graft is attached to the sacral promontory, which has been predissected down to the level of the anterior ligament of the spine (Figure 19.8).

4. Care must be taken to avoid the middle sacral vasculature, and the mesh must be completely reperitonealized in order to avoid problems with adhesive disease that can occur with mesh in the abdomen. The graft should not be placed with tension (Figure 19.9).

COMPLICATIONS AND THEIR PREVENTION

- *Infection*: Mesh should be handled with clean gloves in order to minimize potential infection.
- *Recurrence*: Patients have a tendency to do 'too much' in the postoperative period. Repetitive straining or heavy lifting must be avoided.
- Surgeons who deal with pelvic floor reconstruction must be knowledgeable, versatile, resourceful, and resilient if they are to be successful in treating these pervasive problems.

SUGGESTED READING

- Lyons TL. Minimally invasive retropubic colposuspension. Gynaecol Endosc 1995;4:189–94.
- Ross J. Two techniques of laparoscopic Burch repair for stress incontinence: a prospective, randomized study. J Am Assoc Gynecol Laparosc 1996;3: 351–7.

- Lee CL, Yen CF, Wang CJ, Jain S, Soong YK. Extraperitoneal approach to laparoscopic Burch colposuspension. J Am Assoc Gynecol Laparosc 2001;8:374–7.
- Zullo F, Palomba S, Piccione F, et al. Laparoscopic Burch colposuspension: a randomized controlled trial comparing two transperitoneal surgical techniques. Obstet Gynecol 2001;98:783–8.
- Margossian H, Walters MD, Falcone T. Laparoscopic management of pelvic organ prolapse. Eur J Obstet Gynecol Reprod Biol 1999;85:57–62.

20

Laparoscopic excision of rudimentary uterine horn

Togas Tulandi

Arcuate uterus with a rudimentary uterine horn develops from incomplete atresia of one of the two müllerian ducts during embryogenesis. The rudimentary horn can have a cavity (cavitated) or be noncavitated, and the cavity could be communicating or not communicating with the uterine cavity of the arcuate uterus. In most cases, there is no communication between the uterine cavity proper and the cavity of the rudimentary horn (Figure 20.1). As a result, menstrual blood will accumulate in the rudimentary horn (hematometra), causing cyclic abdominal pain. This also predisposes to the development of endometriosis. The rudimentary horn may be separated from the unicornuate uterus with fibrous tissue or adherent to it.

Pregnancy can be located in the rudimentary uterine horn, usually in the noncommunicating type. However, pregnancy in the rudimentary horn, whether communicating or noncommunicating, carries the risks of uterine rupture. Preconception diagnosis is desirable – this is established by magnetic resonance imaging (MRI). Occasionally, a noncavitated rudimentary horn is misinterpreted as a pedunculated uterine fibroid. A cavitated uterine horn can be easily identified by transvaginal ultrasonography. Noncavitated rudimentary uterine horn is asymptomatic and does not require treatment. In contrast, excision of a cavitated uterine horn is recommended.

PROCEDURE

Excision of the rudimentary horn is similar to that of hysterectomy. The round ligament, the proximal part of the fallopian tube, and the ovarian ligament are electrocoagulated and divided, allowing access to the retroperitoneal space and visualization of the uterine vessels. The bladder peritoneum anterior to the uterine horn is hydrodissected and divided, and the bladder is dissected off the lower part of the uterine horn.

Figures 20.2 and 20.3 show rudimentary uterine horns in a patient with Mayer–Rokitansky–Küster–Hauser (MRKH) syndrome. The two horns are completely separated with a long fibrous band. In this case, mobilization of the bladder was not required.

Separation of the horn from the uterus is easy when there is a band of fibrous tissue between them. The fibrous band can be simply coagulated and divided. The procedure is more complex when the horn is closely attached to the uterus. Separation of the horn can be accomplished with sharp dissection at the point where they join. Hemostasis is done using bipolar coagulation, and the uterine defect is closed with a few sutures.

The excised rudimentary horn is extracted intact through either a colpotomy incision or an extended lateral port. This will allow confirmation of whether the horn is cavitated.

COMPLICATIONS AND THEIR PREVENTION

- Without MRI, the diagnosis can be missed even intraoperatively. Hysteroscopy at best would reveal absence of one tubal ostium, and laparoscopy

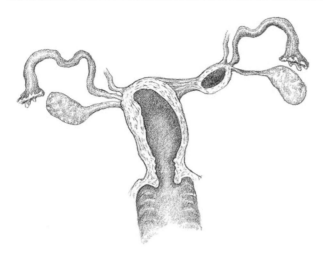

Figure 20.1 The most common type of rudimentary uterine horn – cavitated and noncommunicating. The horn is separated from the unicornuate uterus with a fibrous band.

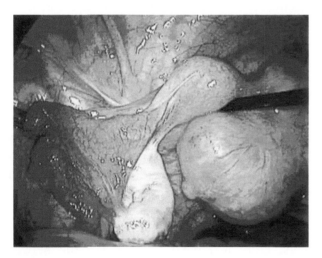

Figure 20.2 Left rudimentary uterine horn with a subserous fibroid in a patient with Mayer–Rokitansky– Küster–Hauser (MRKH) syndrome.

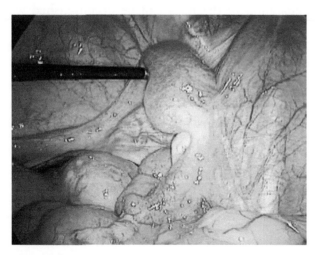

Figure 20.3 Right rudimentary uterine horn in the same patient as in Figure 20.2.

would not provide any indication as far whether the horn is cavitated.

- Associated vaginal malformation, such as obstructed hemivagina, and urinary abnormalities should be ruled out prior to surgery.
- The course of the ureter should be followed. Note that the ureter ipsilateral to the rudimentary horn is often located higher than the opposite side.
- The presence of endometriosis could distort the anatomy.
- The cleavage plane between the uterus proper and the rudimentary horn is ill defined. Hysteroscopic illumination can facilitate identification of the surgical plane
- Myometrial defects on the uterus proper should be sutured thoroughly.
- Due to the risks of ectopic pregnancy secondary to transperitoneal migration of gametes, the surgeon should excise the ipsilateral fallopian tube as well.

CONTRAINDICATIONS

Unlike other conditions, elective operation in a woman who might have a rudimentary uterine horn should not be performed without MRI diagnosis. It is mandatory that the surgeon have expertise in laparoscopic suturing.

SUGGESTED READING

- American Fertility Society. The American Fertility Society classifications of the adnexal adhesions, distal tubal occlusion, tubal occlusion secondary to tubal ligation, tubal pregnancy, mullerian anomalies and intrauterine adhesions. Fertil Steril 1998;49: 944–55.
- Fedele L, Bianchi S, Zanconato G, Berlanda N, Bergamini V. Laparoscopic removal of the cavitated noncommunicating rudimentary uterine horn: surgical aspects in 10 cases. Fertil Steril 2005;83: 432–6.
- Jayasinghe Y, Rane A, Stalewski H, Grover S. The presentation and early diagnosis of the rudimentary uterine horn. Obstet Gynecol 2005; 105:1456–67.

21

Laparoscopy in pregnancy

Togas Tulandi

The incidence of nonobstetric surgery during pregnancy is approximately 1 in 500 pregnancies. The common laparoscopic procedures performed in pregnancy are cholecystectomy, appendectomy, adnexal surgery (Figure 21.1), and management of heterotopic pregnancy. Treatment of pregnant women requires consideration of the well-being of both mother and fetus. Furthermore, diagnosis in pregnancy is complicated by the displacement of organs by the gravid uterus. This can cause delays in intervention, increasing fetal and maternal morbidity.

PROCEDURE

- The set-up is similar to that for laparoscopy in nonpregnant women.
- The patient can be placed in the dorsal lithotomy position in the first half of pregnancy. In the second half of pregnancy, a left lateral position will prevent inferior vena cava compression.
- There is no instrumentation of the cervix or the uterine cavity.
- Determine the height of the uterus.
- Open laparoscopy is the best approach for a uterus of ≥16 weeks' gestational size (Figure 21.2).
- Trocars are inserted supraumbilical, subxiphoid, or at the Palmers point (Figure 21.3).
- Secondary trocars should be inserted higher than the level of the uterine fundus (Figure 21.3).
- Maintain intraabdominal pressure <12 mmHg.
- Reduce operative time to minimize the risk of maternal hypercarbia and fetal acidosis.

- Use of nitrous oxide in anaesthesia is advantageous due to its higher oxygen content.

COMPLICATIONS AND THEIR PREVENTION

- There can be injury to the gravid uterus and the small bowel. Accordingly, for a uterus > 16 weeks' gestational size, the surgeon should insert the Veress needle at the Palmers point or use alternative sites, such as supraumbilical or subxiphoid. We prefer to do open laparoscopy.
- Pneumoperitoneum and increased abdominal pressure cause decrease uterine blood flow, lung compliance, and functional residual capacity. This can be mitigated by maintaining the intraabdominal pressure <12 mmHg, placing the patient in the Trendelenburg and left lateral decubitus position, and using positive-pressure ventilation.
- Rapid carbon dioxide (CO_2) absorption can lead to increased arterial CO_2 pressure and decreased arterial pH. Several measures should be taken, including monitoring of end-tidal volume CO_2 concentration and arterial blood gases, control of maternal hyperventilation, and continuous fetal monitoring. Alternatively, the surgeon can perform gasless laparoscopy. This approach eliminates the effects of CO_2 insufflations and high intraabdominal pressure. However, it is associated with a small intraabdominal space, a decreased operative field, and retraction pain.
- There is a potential risk of exposure to intraabdominal smoke, including carbon monoxide,

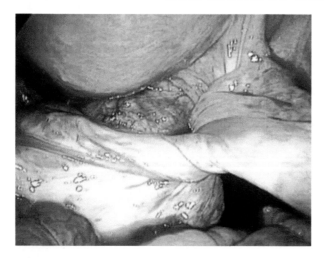

Figure 21.1 Torsion of right adnexa in pregnancy.

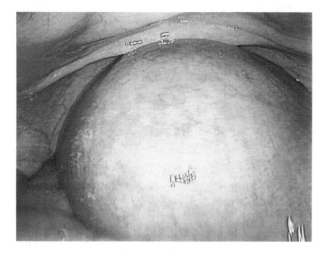

Figure 21.2 Uterus of 16 weeks' gestational size occupying almost the entire pelvic cavity.

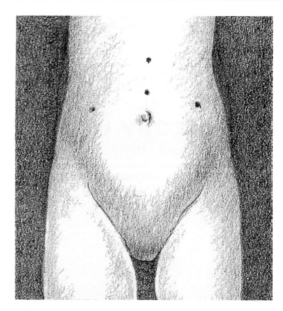

Figure 21.3 Trocar sites for operative laparoscopy in the 2nd trimester of pregnancy.

CONTRAINDICATIONS

The most common gynaecologic indication for surgery in pregnancy is persistent ovarian cyst. In general, surgery can be postponed until the 2nd trimester or until after delivery.

SUGGESTED READING

- Al-Fozan H, Tulandi T. Safety and risks of laparoscopy in pregnancy. Curr Opin Obstet Gynecol 2002; 14:375–9.
- Stepp K, Falcone T. Laparoscopy in the second trimester of pregnancy. Obstet Gynecol Clin North Am 2004;31:485–96.

generated by electrosurgery and laser. Reduction of surgical time and rapid evacuation of smoke during surgery will reduce this risk.
- Performing surgery in the 2 trimester of pregnancy reduces the risks of miscarriage, teratogenicity, and preterm labor.

22

Laparoscopic abdominal cerclage

Togas Tulandi

Cervical incompetence is diagnosed in 0.1–1.0% of all pregnancies and in 8% of women with repeated midtrimester pregnancy loss. The treatment consists of placing a pursestring suture around the cervix. The indications for abdominal cerclage are an extremely short cervix or a deformed, scarred, or absent cervix preventing adequate application of vaginal cerclage. Women who have failed vaginal cerclage are also potential candidates.

Potential advantages of the abdominal approach include high placement of the suture, no slippage of the suture, lack of a foreign body inside the vagina that could predispose to ascending infection and premature labor, and the ability to leave the suture in place between pregnancies. The surgeon can perform abdominal cerclage during pregnancy or in the nonpregnant state.

PROCEDURE

The procedure is performed under general anesthesia. The patient is placed in the dorsal lithotomy position and an indwelling catheter is inserted. In a nonpregnant state, a uterine manipulator is inserted into the uterine cavity. Laparoscopy is performed in the usual fashion, using two secondary trocars in low abdominal quadrants. The surgeon should place these trocars higher than the level of the uterine fundus.

The peritoneum of the uterovesical reflection is injected with normal saline to facilitate separation of the bladder from the cervix (Figure 22.1). We identify but do not dissect the uterine vessels.

Cerclage is done using a 5 mm Mersilene polyester tape that is first prepared by removing the needles from its ends and tapering the ends. The tape is then passed into the pelvis and positioned behind the uterus.

A disposable EndoClose suturing device (Tyco Healthcare, Gosport, UK) is passed into the abdominal cavity suprapubically. Its tip is directed toward the isthmus, medial to the uterine vessels. The cardinal ligament and the cervical body are pierced until the tip is seen at the posterior leaf of the broad ligament just above the insertion of the uterosacral ligament. The end of the tape is grasped with the device, and the device is retracted anteriorly, bringing the tape with it (Figures 22.2–22.5). The procedure is then repeated on the opposite site, bringing the other end of the tape anteriorly. Using two laparoscopic needle-holders, the two ends of the tape are tied anteriorly with a square knot (Figure 22.6). It is secured by another knot. The excess suture material is trimmed. The abdominal cavity is irrigated with normal saline solution and hemostasis is confirmed.

COMPLICATIONS AND THEIR PREVENTION

- Risks of miscarriage can be prevented by performing the cerclage in the nonpregnant state. In patients whose need for abdominal cerclage is clear, performing the procedure in the nonpregnant state has some advantages. These include easy manipulation and exposure, and minimal bleeding.

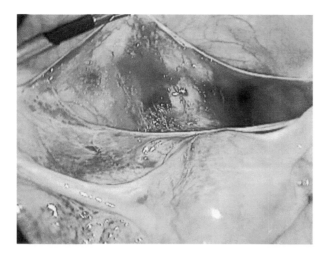

Figure 22.1 The peritoneum of the uterovesical reflection has been separated from the cervix.

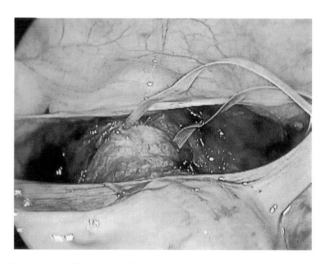

Figure 22.4 Posterior view of the uterus. Both ends of the tape have been pulled anteriorly.

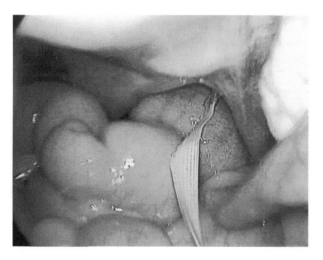

Figure 22.2 An EndoClose device grasps the end of the Mersilene tape behind the uterus.

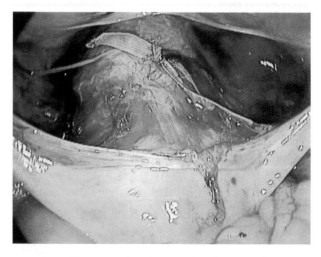

Figure 22.5 The suture has been properly placed.

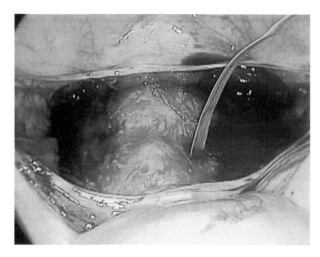

Figure 22.3 The tape has been pulled anteriorly. Note that the uterine vessels are located laterally.

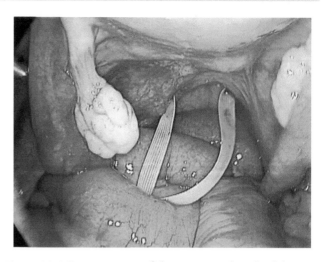

Figure 22.6 The suture has been tied with square knots.

- As dissection of the uterine vessels is not required, the risk of bleeding is minimal.
- An enlarged uterus complicates placement of the device. Ideally, the procedure should be performed at or before 13 weeks of gestation.
- The possibility of infection is decreased by the administration of prophylactic antibiotics.

CONTRAINDICATIONS

Contraindications to abdominal cerclage are similar to those to the vaginal approach (ruptured membranes, intrauterine infections, etc.). A uterus of more than 13 weeks' gestational size might lead to failure of laparoscopic cerclage. Familiarity with laparoscopic intracorporeal knot tying is mandatory.

SUGGESTED READING

- Gallot D, Savary D, Laurichesse H, et al. Experience with three cases of laparoscopic trans-abdominal cervico-isthmic cerclage ad two subsequent pregnancies. BJOG 2003;110:696–700.
- Mingione M, Scibetta J, Sanko S, Phipps W. Clinical outcomes following interval laparoscopic trans-abdominal cerclage placement: case series. Hum Reprod 2003;18:1716–19.
- Al-Fadhli R, Tulandi T. Laparoscopic abdominal cerclage. Obstet Gynecol Clin North Am 2004; 31:497–504.

23

Laparoscopy in the pediatric and adolescent population

Suketu M Mansuria and Joseph S Sanfilippo

The use of laparoscopy by gynecologists in treating pediatric and adolescent patients is relatively new. This chapter will discuss the preoperative considerations, set-up, and techniques unique to this population. Although laparoscopy has a myriad of indications, in this chapter we will concentrate on the management of pelvic pain/endometriosis and adnexal masses. Indications and techniques for incidental appendectomy will also be presented.

PREOPERATIVE CONSIDERATIONS

Many of the same considerations that are taken into account when deciding to operate on an adult come into play when deciding to operate on a child.

Laparoscopy is generally contraindicated in hemodynamically unstable patients or in patients with a known history of severe adhesive disease. Also, patients with pulmonary or cardiac compromise may not tolerate the increased intraabdominal pressure of CO_2 insufflation or the Trendelenburg position. The latter compress the vena cava and compromises venous return and decreases diaphragmatic excursion and functional residual capacity.

Pediatric and adolescent patients have elastic abdominal walls, allowing many procedures to be performed through small minilaparotomy incisions. Once the small incision is made, it can be stretched to provide a disproportionately larger area of exposure than a similar incision in adults. Approaching the procedure through a minilaparotomy may allow it to be completed in a short time and reduces the complications associated with longer procedure times.

PREOPERATIVE SET-UP

Procedures can be performed with 5 or 10 mm scopes, but 2 mm endoscopes are available for use in patients.

In patients who are large enough, Allen stirrups should be used for positioning to allow unencumbered access to the vagina during the procedure.

In patients with intact hymens, prepping the vagina can be accomplished with minimal trauma to the hymen using a large 60 cm^3 syringe. The syringe is filled with the prep solution, and the vagina is thoroughly irrigated by introducing the solution into the introitus. This avoids the use of sponges, which can traumatize the hymen during insertion and causes abrasions to the delicate vaginal mucosa during scrubbing.

The use of a uterine manipulator is usually avoided because most are too large for the small uterus in this population. Simple manipulation can also be accomplished with the help of an assistant who inserts one finger gently into the posterior fornix and elevates the uterus intraoperatively with gentle upward pressure. If a uterine manipulator is absolutely necessary, a small cervical dilator can be advanced into the cavity and secured to a cervical tenaculum, allowing for basic uterine manipulation.

Tucking the arms

Tucking the patient's arms by their side during the procedure is useful. Given the children's small stature, the shorter distance between outstretched arms and the pelvis limits the surgeon's maneuverability, and by tucking the arms, the surgeon is able to more ergonomically position himself or herself above the level of the shoulders. This is also a safety precaution, because inadvertently leaning on an outstretched arm of a small patient can have dire consequences. The arms are tucked by first wrapping the entire arm in egg crate and then securing the arms against their sides with the help of bed sheets (Figure 23.1). The fingers should be protected so that they are not injured during articulation of the foot of the bed or the stirrups, and the arms should be placed at the patient's side in their normal, anatomic position in order to reduce the risk of a median nerve injury.

Entry into the abdominal cavity

Abdominal entry can be accomplished with either a Veress needle or by an open technique. The distance between the anterior abdominal wall and abdominal aorta is often short; thus, an open technique that allows entry into the abdomen layer by layer reduces the risk of vascular injury. Also, young patients have very elastic tissue, which can make confirmation of intraabdominal placement of the Veress needle deceptive.

Entry through a vertical incision centered at the midpoint of the patient's umbilicus is recommended. This not only has cosmetic benefits, as the scar is hidden completely within the umbilicus, but also is the thinnest portion of the anterior abdominal wall, facilitates entry easiest.

Pneumoperitoneum

The total volume of gas to be introduced to establish pneumoperitoneum is variable. This variability is mainly due to the fact that the physiologic changes (i.e., alterations in cardiac output, diaphragmatic excursion, pulmonary functional residual capacity, and renal blood flow) associated with pneumoperitoneum are directly related to the increase in intraabdominal pressure, not to the volume of gas introduced. Patient size, abdominal wall distensibility, and amount of muscle relaxation also play an important role in determining intraabdominal pressure. Therefore,

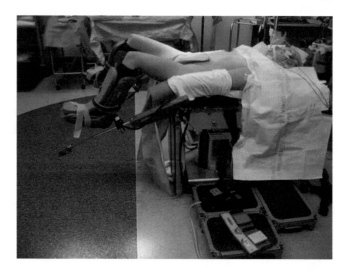

Figure 23.1 Properly positioned patient with legs in Allen stirrups and arms tucked.

it is preferable to set the pressure limit on pressure regulated automatic insufflators. For infants, the pressure is set at 6–8 mmHg. For children, most procedures can be accomplished using pressures of 8–10 mmHg, with an increase to 12–15 mmHg for older, larger children. These pressures are only general guidelines, as the patient's medical condition may dictate lower pressures.

When placing primary and secondary trocars, transiently insufflating the abdomen to a pressure of 25 mmHg prevents tenting of the anterior abdominal wall during trocar insertion and increases the distance between the trocar entry site and the underlying bowel and vasculature (Figure 23.2). Once the trocars are inserted, the pressure is reduced to what will be used during the case.

Secondary trocars

Prior to placing lateral lower abdominal ports, the inferior epigastric vessels should be identified bilaterally. The medial umbilical ligaments (also known as the obliterated umbilical arteries) can be used as landmarks. The inferior epigastric vessels are invariably located just lateral to these ligaments (Figure 23.3).

Securing the trocars in place can also be difficult. Screwtype trocars often tear the delicate skin of children and may slip out during the proceedute due to the lack of 'grip' provided by thin abdominal walls. Traditional trocars can be sutured into place, and trocars with expandable flanges, such as Pediports

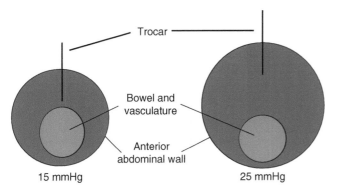

Figure 23.2 Transiently increasing the insufflation pressure to 25 mmHg prior to trocar insertion increases the distance between the trocar and underlying bowel and vasculature.

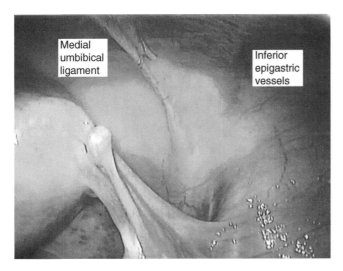

Figure 23.3 Relationship of the inferior epigastric vessels to the medial umbilical ligament on the right side. Note that the vessels are lateral to the ligament.

(US Surgical, Norwalk, CT), prevents slippage. In older children, where sheath length is not as much of an issue, Versa-Step (US Surgical) trocars can be used. These trocars dilate the fascial defect instead of cutting it. The dilating action, along with a textured sheath, provides adequate resistance to slippage (Figure 23.4).

All trocar sites in children, regardless of the size, should be sutured in order to prevent hernias. Children's fascia is not as strong as that of adults; therefore, fascial defects due to trocars can expand from manipulation of the trocar introperatively and lead to a substantially larger defect. Herniation through trocar sites less than 10 mm has been reported.

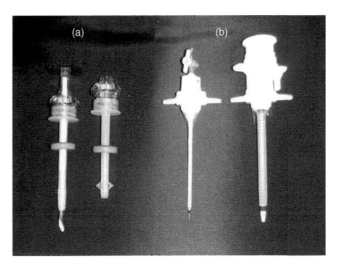

Figure 23.4 (a) Pediport trocars (US Surgical, Norwalk, CT) with the expandable flange retracted and deployed. (b) Versa-step trocars (US Surgical) with Veress needle and unexpanded sheath and dilating blunt trocar and expanded sheath.

CHRONIC PELVIC PAIN/ENDOMETRIOSIS

Table 23.1 lists some common causes of chronic pelvic pain in the adolescent population. This section will deal with chronic pelvic pain secondary to endometriosis.

The true incidence of endometriosis in this age group is unknown. It is estimated to range from 19% to 65% in teens with chronic pelvic pain. Pelvic pain, with or without dysmenorrhea, is often the presenting complaint, and the pain is usually refractory to nonsteridal anti-inflammatory drugs and oral contraceptive pills. Infertility and pelvic masses (i.e., endometriomas) are rarely seen in this age group. Physical findings of nodularity and fixed uteri are rare in adolescents, and their examination usually only reveals moderate tenderness.[1]

Endometriotic implants in adolescents have a different appearance from those seen in adults (Figure 23.5). This may be secondary to the natural life cycle of endometriosis, with the implants seen in adolescents being of the early variety whereas the classic lesion seen in adults is the blue-black, powder-burn lesion. Adolescents' lesions take on a more atypical appearance. The most common appearance is that of red 'flame' petechial lesions, but clear and white lesions are also seen. Vesicles are also a common lesion type in adolescent patients.[2]

Treatment consists of excision or fulguration, with excision being favored for two reasons. Excision

Table 23.1 Causes of chronic pelvic pain in the adolescent population

Reproductive system
Chronic pelvic inflammatory disease
Endometriosis
Adhesions
Ovarian neoplasia
Intermittent ovarian torsion
Primary dysmenorrhea
Outflow tract obstruction (i.e., müllerian anomaly)
Gastrointestinal tract
Irritable bowel syndrome
Inflammatory bowel disease (i.e., Crohn's disease or ulcerative colitis)
Constipation
Hernia
Recurrent appendiceal colic
Recurrent partial small bowel obstruction
Musculoskeletal
Scoliosis and kyphosis
Myofascial syndrome
Strains/sprains
Spine injuries
Systemic disease
Acute intermittent porphyria
Lymphoma
Heavy metal poisoning
Neurofibromatosis
Other
Abuse
Psychosocial stress
Psychiatric disorder

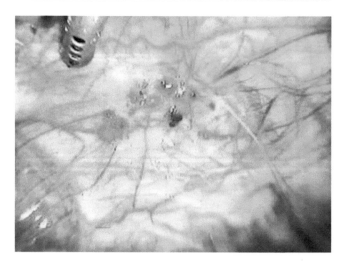

Figure 23.5 Characteristic endometriotic lesion in an adolescent patient. The lesion is red and vesicular.

diagnosis to be made. It also does not take into account the depth of the lesion. Often the portion of the lesion that is visible to the surgeon is just the 'tip of the iceberg'. By fulgurating the lesion, deeper portions of the endometriosis may go untreated. Excision allows for the entire lesion to be removed in its entirety.

When treating lesions, the surgeon at all times must be cognizant of the location of the ureters, rectum, and uterine arteries. Ureteric stents and rectal probes can be utilized to help demarcate these structures. Also, lesions should be pulled away from the sidewall prior to treatment in order to reduce the risk of injury to underlying tissue.

ADNEXAL MASSES

The differential diagnosis is quite long and may involve organ systems that are not usually dealt with by gynecologists (Table 23.2).

The most common presenting symptom is abdominal pain, which is found in up to 70% of patients.[3] The majority of patients will also have a palpable mass on examination.

The work-up for these masses should include imaging of the pelvis, usually by ultrasound.

Characteristics on ultrasound that would increase the suspicion for a malignancy include solid masses, excrescences or nodules within the mass, septations,

allows the removed tissue to be evaluated histopathologically. Pathologic confirmation of endometriosis is especially important as it allows the clinician to tailor future treatment and work-ups appropriately. Visual diagnosis of endometriosis has been shown to have poor positive and negative predictive values. The poor predictive value of visual diagnosis is further worsened by the atypical lesions seen in this population. Fulguration does not allow for a tissue and decreased resistive indices.[4] When a malignancy of the ovary is suspected, tumor markers may be helpful in making the diagnosis.

In a retrospective study of 140 females aged between 2 days and 21 years who underwent operative intervention for an ovarian mass, ovarian cysts were the most common abnormality found. Overall, 57.9% of these patients had some form of benign ovarian cyst, such as a corpus luteal cyst, a follicular cyst, a paratubal or paraovarian cyst, or a neonatal cyst. Dermoids and benign ovarian tumors were the next most common masses (30%). Malignancy was seen in 11 patients (7.8%), and the malignancy rate was higher in those patients under the age of 15.[3]

Operative intervention is warranted if torsion is suspected, in the unstable patient with adnexal mass, or when there is a suspicion of malignancy or the mass is persistent.

When malignancy is not suspected, large cysts can be managed laparoscopically by decompressing them prior to performing any additional procedures. Decompression is best performed by making a small puncture into the cyst and then inserting a suction–irrigator through the hole and aspirating all of the fluid. After decompressing the cyst, the surgeon can proceed with a complete cystectomy.

Laparoscopic cystectomy is best performed using a combination of traction–countertraction and aqua dissection. Traction is applied to the cyst wall as blunt dissection separates the cyst from the ovary. Aqua dissection is performed by inserting the tip of the suction–irrigator between the ovary and cyst and then using the pressurized flow of fluid to displace tissue and create natural cleavage planes along the path of least resistance.

Conservative ovarian surgery is desirable, but in certain circumstances salpingo-oophorectomy is indicated. Salpingo-oophorectmy is performed in the same manner as in adult patients.

In many situations, the fallopian tube can be spared. Often, enlargement of the ovary elongates the meso-ovarium, allowing oophorectomy to be performed by coming across and controlling the meso-ovarium and avoiding the infundibulopelvic ligament. This approach has the added benefits of decreasing the risk of injuring the ureter by controlling the vasculature (i.e., the meso-ovarium) more lateral than in a traditional salpingo-oophorectomy (i.e., infundibulopelvic ligament)

Table 23.2 Differential diagnoses of adnexal masses

Ovarian functional cyst
Paraovarian/paratubal cyst
Ovarian tumor – benign or malignant
Hydrosalpinx
Leiomyoma
Peri-appendiceal abscess
Ectopic pregnancy
Hematometra
Urachal cyst
Mesenteric cyst
Pelvic kidney
Hydronephrosis
Wilms' tumor
Neuroblastoma
Tubo-ovarian abscess
Bowel duplication

and impairing future fertility to a lesser degree by preserving the fallopian tube.

APPENDECTOMY

The decision to perform an incidental appendectomy is based on the premise that the appendix is a vestigial, functionless organ, with the potential only to contribute to pathologic change. However, some physicians have hypothesized that the lymphoid tissue of the appendix exerts a protective function against virus and tumor antigens. This view has been refuted by well-designed studies demonstrating no apparent predisposition to cancer in those patients who have had an appendectomy.[5]

The lifetime risk for appendicitis in females is 6.7%, and the highest incidence of appendicitis is found in persons aged 10–19 years.

Incidental appendectomy is a relatively safe procedure that adds minimal to no morbidity when performed during another procedure, and does not increase the wound infection rate, incidence of sepsis, or length of hospital stay.

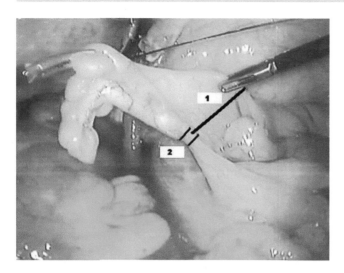

Figure 23.6 Normal appendix. 1. Level at which the mesoappendix and appendiceal artery should be ligated. 2. Level at which the appendix should be transected.

Appendectomy may play a role in treatment of patients with chronic pelvic pain. It has been shown that appendices removed during surgery for chronic pelvic pain have a high incidence of pathology and that patients report significant pain improvement.[6]

Appendectomies can be performed by a myriad of different techniques. Surgical clips, linear stapling devices, bipolar cautery, or endoscopic loops can all be used.

The basic steps are as follows. First, the appendix must be localized and freed from any adhesions. Lysis of adhesions continues until the junction between the appendix and cecum is clearly identified. Second, the blood supply of the appendix, namely the appendiceal artery, must be secured. This vessel courses through the mesoappendix. Once the mesoappendix has been ligated and cut, the appendix can be removed. This is usually performed with a linear stapling device or endoscopic loops (Figure 23.6). After the appendix has been removed, the surgical field is copiously irrigated.

Care must be taken to excise the appendix as close to the appendiceal–cecal junction as possible in order to avoid leaving a large stump.

SUGGESTED READING

- Sanfilippo JS, Schroeder B. Pelvic pain in children and adolescents. In: Carpenter SEK, Rock JA, eds. Pediatric and Adolescent Gynecology, 2nd ed, Philedelphia: Lippincott Williams & Wilkins, 2000:287–9.
- Laufer MR, Goldstein DP. Dysmenorrhea, pelvic pain, and the premenstrual syndrome. In: Emans SJ, Laufer MR, Goldstein DP, eds. Pediatric and Adolescent Gynecology. Philedelphia: Lippincott-Raven, 1998: 363–410.
- Templeman C, Fallat M, Blinchevsky A, Hertweck S. Noninflammatory ovarian masses in girls and young women. Obstet Gynecol 2000;96:229–33.
- Brown D. Sonographic differentiation of benign versus malignant adnexal masses. UpToDate, 2004. http://www.uptodate.com.
- Moertel CG, Nobrega FT, Elveback LR, Wentz JR. A prospective study of appendectomy and predisposition to cancer. Surg Gynecol Obstet 1974;138: 549–53.
- AlSalilli M, Vilos GA. Prospective evaluation of laparoscopic appendectomy in women with chronic right lower quadrant pain. J Am Assoc Gynecol Laparosc 1995;2:139–42.

24

Transvaginal laparoscopy

S Gordts

Transvaginal endoscopic exploration is intended to make exploration of the female internal organs as minimally invasive as possible without compromising the diagnostic accuracy of the investigation. It allows direct and easy access and visualization of the tubo-ovarian structures without supplementary manipulation. With the endoscope in the same axis as the tubo-ovarian structures, the total ovarian surface and the fossa ovarica can easily be accessed. In the absence of any manipulation, transvaginal laparoscopy allows inspection of different structures in their normal position and normal relation to each other. This allows direct observation of normal physiologic events at ovulation and ovum pickup. (Figure 24.1). Compared with standard laparoscopy, following this procedure most patients had minimal pain (mainly in the lower abdomen).

TECHNIQUE AND INSTRUMENTS

Access to the pouch of Douglas is gained through a needle puncture of the posterior fornix using a specially developed needle–trocar system. The access trocar consists of three parts: (a) a spring-loaded needle, (b) a dilating device, and (c) an outer trocar (Figure 24.2). The spring-loaded needle enables rapid access to the pouch of Douglas. The length of the loaded needle can be preset between 1 cm and 2.5 cm. In general, we use a preset depth of 1.5 cm. The endoscope used is a 2.9 mm endoscope with a 30° angled optical lens – the same as for hysteroscopy. The outer trocar diameter is 3.4 mm (Figure 24.3).

With the patient in a dorsal decubitus position, the posterior lip of the cervix is grasped and lifted with forceps. The assembled needle is placed at the posterior fornix on the midline about 1.5 cm under the cervix. Up-and-down movements with the forceps will clearly show the bulging of the vaginal fornix, which is helpful in identifying the point of entrance. After the spring-loaded needle has been placed at the correct point, it is released.

While pushing the dilating sheet and the outer trocar gently forward, the needle is slowly withdrawn and the site of entrance is dilated up to the diameter of the outer trocar (4 mm). The endoscope is introduced and correct intraabdominal localization is confirmed.

DIAGNOSTIC TRANSVAGINAL LAPAROSCOPY

The posterior site of the uterus is examined and, in the absence of a panoramic view, serves as a landmark. During the entire procedure, we use a continuous flow of prewarmed Ringer's lactate; in general not exceeding 500 cm^3. This distention medium keeps the organs afloat and enables accurate visualization of lesions on the surfaces of tubes and ovaries (Figure 24.4).

While inspecting the fimbriae, salpingoscopy and (when indicated) a patency test with methylene blue can be performed (Figure 24.5). At the end of the procedure, the endoscope is removed, and the distending solution is allowed to escape through the

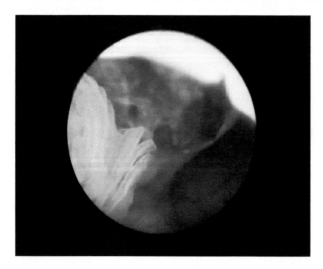

Figure 24.1 Allowing inspection of the tubo-ovarian organs in their natural position, transvaginal laparoscopy offers the possibility of evaluation of the events occurring at the moment of ovum release. The erected fimbriae are in close contact with the ovulatory ostium.

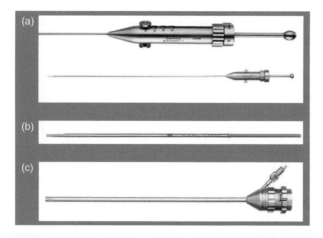

Figure 24.2 A specially developed needle–trocar system consists out of three parts: (a) a spring-loaded needle (with a close-up of the spring-load mechanism); (b) a dilating trocar; (c) an outer trocar. The spring-load system allows rapid access to the pouch of Douglas. (Karl Storz, Tuttlingen, Germany.)

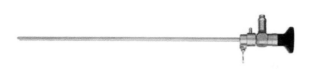

Figure 24.3 The 30°angled 2.9 mm endoscope with 3.4 mm diagnostic trocar. (Karl Storz, Tuttlingen, Germany.)

cannula before withdrawal. There is no need to suture the puncture site, unless there is active bleeding.

OPERATIVE PROCEDURES

In the absence of a panoramic view, transvaginal laparoscopy is not designed for acute conditions such as intraperitoneal bleeding or infection. However, it offers an accurate detection of subtle lesions on peritoneal and ovarian surfaces (Figure 24.6). The transvaginal operative route is particularly useful in the treatment of minimal or mild peritoneal and ovarian endometriosis and for surgical treatment of clomiphene-resistant polycystic ovarian syndrome. We conduct operative interventions under general anesthesia or sedation in an ambulatory center.

Instruments

For operative procedures, the endoscope is fitted in an outer operative sheet of 5 mm with one working-channel instrument or in a 6.5 mm outer trocar with the possibility of two working channels (Figure 24.7).

All 5 Fr instruments, including scissors and grasping and biopsy forceps, can be used. Cutting and coagulation are performed using a bipolar needle and bipolar probe.

Endometriosis

All structures preferentially affected by endometriosis are directly accessible by the transvaginal route: the posterior leaf of the broad ligament, the posterior side of the uterus, and the uterosacral ligament. Surgery is limited to stage I and II endometriosis.

Endometriotic cysts can also be treated. The most appropriate route of access is through an opening at the site of invagination. With transvaginal laparoscopy, the site is located at the anterolateral site of the ovary. It is easily accessible without supplementary manipulation. We first liberate adhesions at the fossa ovarica. A wide opening is created at the site of inversion; this is followed by a superficial coagulation of the endometriotic implants. In contrast to other benign ovarian cysts, the wall of an endometrioma does not collapse. After rinsing and aspiration of the contents of the cyst, endometriotic implants and neovascularization will be seen in the cyst wall. A biopsy is taken, and

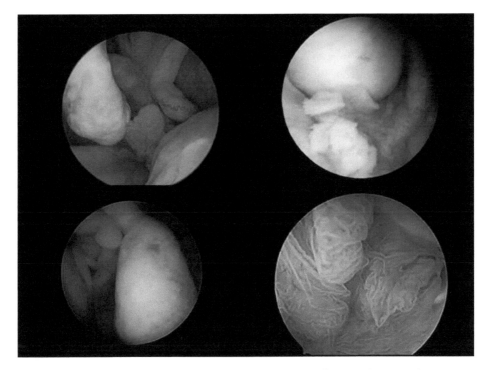

Figure 24.4 The use of Ringer's lactate as distention medium keeps the organs afloat. Without supplementary manipulation, tubo-ovarian structures can be inspected accurately in their normal position.

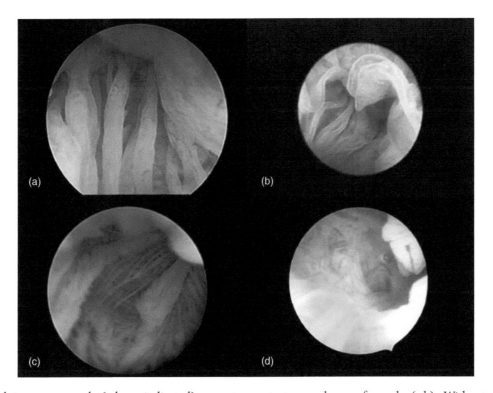

Figure 24.5 Salpingoscopy and (when indicated) a patency test can be performed. (a,b) Without supplementary manipulation, salpingoscopy is possible in 50% of the attempted tubes. (c,d) Salpingoscopy in a hypoplastic tube showing (c) transparency of the tubal wall and thinning of the mucosal folds and (d) the presence of intratubal adhesions.

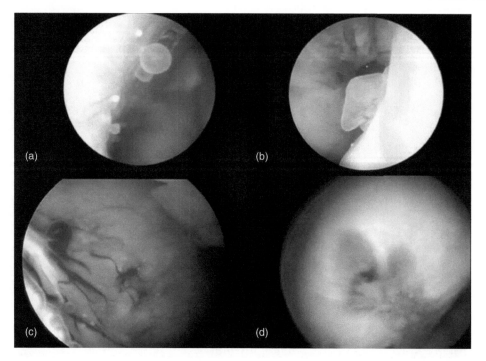

Figure 24.6 Subtle lesions upon the peritoneal and ovarian surface are clearly visible with transvaginal laparoscopy using a watery distention medium: (a) vesicular peritoneal lesion; (b) papillary endometriotic lesion; (c) hemorrhagic endometriotic lesion with neoangiogenesis; (d) endometriotic ovarian lesion covered by adhesions.

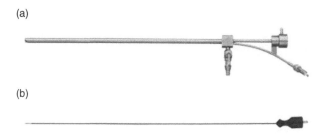

Figure 24.7 Minimally invasive operative procedures are possible with transvaginal laparoscopy. For this purpose, a one- or two-channel operative trocar is used, allowing the insertion of 5 Fr instruments (a). As prewarmed Ringer's lactate is used as distention medium, bipolar current is mandatory for coagulation and cutting. The 5 Fr bipolar needle is of particular use for drilling of the ovarian capsule (b). (Karl Storz, Tuttlingen, Germany).

the implants are cauterized with bipolar cautery (Figure 24.8).

Ovarian drilling

We use a 5 Fr bipolar needle. The entire ovarian surface can easily be seen. The intestines are kept out of the way by the distending medium and the floating of the organs. The bipolar needle is gently pushed against and perpendicular to the ovarian capsule

(Figure 24.9a). Current is activated with an energy output of 70 W. During activation of the current and to obtain a maximal effect of the energy, inflow of Ringer's lactate is stopped. The needle is easy inserted in the ovarian tissue to a depth of 0.8 cm. We make approximately 10 holes on each ovarian surface, preferentially at the anterolateral site (Figure 24.9b). As prophylactic antibiotic, patients receive 1 g of amoxicillin preoperatively.

POTENTIAL COMPLICATIONS AND THEIR PREVENTION

Entry failure

Our failure rate of access is 3.4%. The use of the small-diameter cannula and the combined needle–trocar system add to the safety of the transvaginal technique.

Needle injury

- Some minor complications can been encountered, including bleeding from the vaginal insertion site, puncture of the posterior uterine wall, and

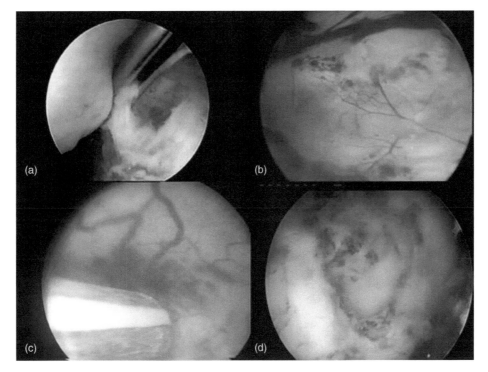

Figure 24.8 Ovarian endometriosis. (a) After removal of superficial adhesions on the ovarian surface, endometriotic implants are identified at the base of the invaginating cyst. (b) In the absence of high intraabdominal pressure, neoangiogenesis is clearly visible. (c) Bipolar coagulation of the endometriotic implants with a 5 Fr bipolar probe (Karl Storz, Tuttlinger, Germany). (d) View after coagulation of the inner lining of the endometriotic cyst with the bipolar coagulation probe. In contrast with other benign ovarian cysts, there is no collapse of the rigid cyste wall.

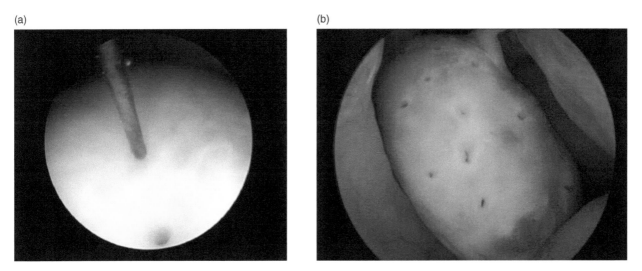

Figure 24.9 Drilling of ovarian capsule: (a) the bipolar needle is placed perpendicular to the ovarian surface; (b) the presence of small holes on the ovarian surface after drilling.

needle perforation of the rectum with no sequellae (0.7%).

- Rectal perforation could be a potentially serious complication. However, generally bowel injuries are recognized during the procedure and nonleaking injury can be managed expectantly without consequences. Routine vaginal examination and vaginal ultrasound to exclude pathology of the pouch of Douglas should be done before the procedure. Patients with narrow vagina, fixed and retroverted uterus, obliterated cul-de-sac, and indurated posterior cervix should not undergo this procedure. In addition, acute clinical conditions or large ovarian cysts are absolute contraindications to the transvaginal approach.

Injury during ovarian drilling

Misidentification of the surface of the intestine as the ovarian surface has led to transvaginal drilling of the intestinal wall. The intestines can be kept away by filling up the abdomen with a sufficient volume of Ringer's lactate ($\geq 300\,\text{ml}$). The ability of the surgeon to recognize different organs on transvaginal laparoscopy is mandatory.

SUGGESTED READING

- Gordts S, Puttemans P, Gordts S, Brosens I, Campo R. Transvaginal hydrolaparoscopy. Best Pract Res Clin Obst Gynaecol 2005;19:757–67.

- Verhoeven HC, Gordts S, Campo R, Puttemans P, Brosens I. Role of transvaginal laparoscopy in the investigation of female infertility: a review of 1000 procedures. Gynecol Surg 2004;1:191–3.
- Gordts S, Watrelot A, Campo R, et al. Risk and outcome of bowel injury during transvaginal pelvic endoscopy. Fertil Steril 2001;76:1238–41.
- Gordts S, Puttemans P, Gordts SY, et al. Transvaginal endoscopy and electrocautery of the ovarian capsule in PCO patients. Fertil Steril 2006;86(Suppl 2): S462.
- Chiesa-Montadou S, Rongieres C, Garbin O, Nisand I. About two complications of ovarian drilling by fertiloscopy. Gynecol Obstet Fertil 2003;31:844–6.

25

Endoscopic feto-placental surgery

Tim Van Mieghem, Liesbeth Lewi, Dominique Van Schoubroeck, Roland Devlieger, Luc De Catte and Jan Deprest

The development of high-quality ultrasound equipment and the integration of ultrasound screening in routine prenatal care have increased the detection rate of fetal disorders. Some of these disorders are progressive during intrauterine life and may lead to intrauterine fetal death or irreversible organ damage. In such cases, one could consider treatment during the prenatal period, which addresses the most critical problems until final therapy after birth can be achieved. To qualify for intra-uterine intervention the pathology should be identifiable prenatally, the natural history of the disease should be well documented, and the condition should have a poor outcome when treated postnatally. Moreover, in-utero therapy must be able to reverse or at least to stop the deleterious effect with a minimal maternal risk.

Open fetal surgery such as for resection of a lung lobe or for closing a neural tube defect is rarely required. These procedures carry a risk of fetal mortality and neonatal morbidity due to preterm labour or persistent oligohydramnios. Advances in minimally invasive surgery have allowed performance of procedures by fetoscopy. These are associated with a smaller uterine incision, and would theoretically cause less preterm labour, fewer ruptured membranes, and lower maternal morbidity.

INSTRUMENTS IN OPERATIVE FETOSCOPY

Scopes

Modern fetoscopes are different from their hysteroscopic and laparoscopic counterparts. They have a 'deported eyepiece', thus moving the eyepiece – with a heavy camera connected to it – away from the operator's hand (Figure 25.1). This allows easy and precise handling of the scope – similar to the needling procedures with which fetal medicine specialists are accustomed.

Another characteristic of fetoscopes is their small outer diameter. Most fetoscopes are fiberscopes $\leq 2\,mm$ in diameter. The advantage of using fibers for image and light transmission is that they allow longer instruments. Further, the scopes are semiflexible, which is useful when operating on the anterior side of the uterus.

Sheaths, cannulas, and trocars

For fetoscopic surgery, the scope is housed in a sheath with three major functions. First, in fiberscopes, the sheath is used to determine the curvature of the scope. Second, it serves to irrigate the operative field, providing a clearer view and preventing amniotic debris from adhering to the scope or the laser fiber. We irrigate with warmed Hartmann's solution, passed through a 'hot-line' as used for blood transfusions or a purpose-designed amnio-irrigator. Lastly, sheaths can accommodate instruments, such as forceps or scissors, catheters, and laser fibers.

The scope is inserted through the anterior uterine wall in an area free of placenta and directed toward the operative field. Most procedures can be performed through percutaneous access to the amniotic cavity under local or locoregional anesthesia (Figure 25.2). However, in rare cases of a very large anterior placenta, a minilaparotomy or, more recently, a laparoscopically assisted technique is required. This is to expose the uterus and to allow fundal access without the risk of bowel injury.

Insertion technique

Different techniques of scope insertion can be used. The typical fetoscopic sheath can be advanced directly

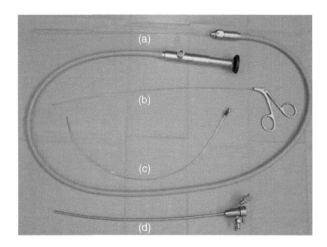

Figure 25.1 Selection of instruments for fetoscopic endotracheal occlusion: (a) 1.2 mm fiberscope with 'deported eyepiece'; (b) 1 mm forceps; (c) needle; (d) curved sheath with working channel.

into the uterus – for this purpose, it is first loaded with a stabbing device (the trocar). After withdrawal of the trocar, the scope is introduced through the actual sheath. This technique has a disadvantage that when advancing or drawing back the sheath, direct friction with the uterine wall and the membranes occurs, which can result in membrane dissociation.

For lengthy procedures or those necessitating scope withdrawal and reinsertion, we use cannulas. This allows free movement and withdrawal of the scope without losing access. This method is more practical.

Twin-video system and operative setup

The image of the operative field (conducted by the scope and a high-quality video camera) is projected on to a television screen. As the fetoscopic image is restricted in depth and width, ultrasound guidance is essential to overview the entire operative field. We use a 'twin-video' system to allow simultaneous projection of endoscopic and ultrasound images on the screen.

The surgeon decides about the relative proportion and position of each image on the screen. The setup of the operating theatre is similar to that for other endoscopic procedures (Figure 25.3).

(a)

(b)

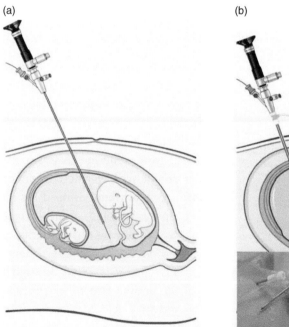
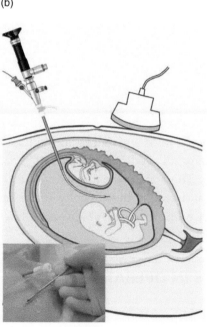

Figure 25.2 (a) Schematic drawing of fetoscopic laser coagulation, in the case of a posterior placenta, using direct insertion of the scope through the sheath – hence without cannula. (b) The case of an anterior placenta, with the use of a curved sheath and flexible cannula (insert). (Drawings K Dalkowski; reprinted with permission of Endopress Karl Storz.)

Additional instruments

We use different instruments for fetal surgery. The most commonly used are thin (400–600 μm diameter) laser fibers that deliver neodymium : yttrium aluminum garnet (Nd:YAG) or diode laser-light to the operating field. Electrosurgery (bipolar forceps) is used to coagulate the umbilical cord in selective fetocide.

FETOSCOPIC COAGULATION OF PLACENTAL VASCULAR ANASTOMOSES.

About one in three twin pregnancies is monozygotic. The longer the period between fertilization and splitting, the more structures both twins have in common. Identical twins who share a placenta – the so-called monochorionic (MC) twins – are most at risk. One of the complications is the twin-to-twin transfusion syndrome (TTTS), which occurs in 5–15% of MC twins. This is an acute pregnancy complication and obstetric emergency, usually occuring between 16 and 26 weeks of pregnancy. When left untreated, TTTS has a perinatal mortality rate of up to 90% and carries a high risk of brain damage in survivors.

One of the treatments of TTTS is *serial amniore-duction* – repeated drainage of large volumes of amniotic fluid under ultrasound guidance. This procedure prevents preterm labor and rupture of the membranes due to polyhydramnios. It also leads to improved uteroplacental circulation and improved fetal hemodynamics. However, in the presence of single intrauterine fetal death (IUFD), the co-twin is at risk of exsanguination. In addition, the decreasing intrauterine pressure after drainage makes the placenta thick – again promoting rapid and major blood and fluid transfer from mother and fetuses into the placenta. The fetuses can become hypovolemic and hypotensive, which may cause brain damage.

Fetoscopic laser coagulation of the placental vascular anastomoses acts directly on the angioarchitecture. It is the treatment of choice between 16 and 26 weeks of pregnancy.

Procedure

- The treatment is performed percutaneously under local or regional anesthesia and with prophylactic antibiotic coverage. An endoscopic cannula is inserted under ultrasound guidance into the amniotic cavity of the recipient, and the vascular equator between the two twins is inspected. Reference points inside the amniotic cavity are both cord insertions and the intertwin membrane. Arteries can be recognized as they cross over the veins and have a darker aspect (deoxygenated blood) (Figure 25.4).

- All visible vascular anastomoses are coagulated over a distance of 1–2 cm by laser energy using a nontouch technique. The fetoscopic intervention is ended with drainage of excessive fluid (until a dynamic venous pressure of 60 mmHg is reached).

- Postoperatively, the patient is observed for surgical complications, with ultrasound imaging to document fetal viability, amniotic fluid volume, resolution of TTTS, and the development of procedure-related complications.

Complications and their prevention

Several short-term complications have been reported after laser coagulation.

- *Preterm prelabor rupture of the membranes (PPROM)* is a complication of any invasive intervention, and occurs in 12% of cases within 3 weeks after the surgery. Early postoperative PPROM can be treated by 'amniopatching'. The intention of this procedure is to close the membrane defect with a fibrin or 'white' blood

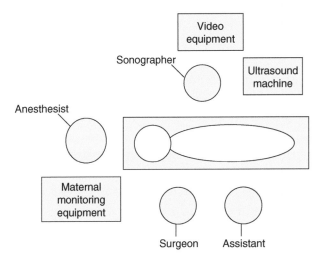

Figure 25.3 Setup of the operating room for in utero sono-endoscopic surgery.

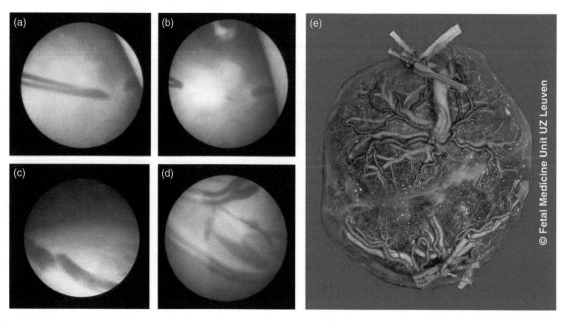

Figure 25.4 (a) Arteriovenous anastomosis at the time of inspection. (b) Arteriovenous anastomosis during coagulation. (c) Arterio-arterial anastomosis. (d) Vessels crossing the membranes – this is not necessarily where they anastomose. (e) Injected placenta after successful laser treatment.

clot generated by the intraamniotic injection of platelets and plasma clotting factors.

- *Prematurity* is a common problem affecting monochorionic twin pregnancies. The risk is higher in the presence of TTTS.
- A relatively frequent complication is the *anemia–polycythemia sequence*, which occurs when a specific pattern of small anastomoses persists. Large arteriovenous anastomoses may result in recurrent or reversal of TTTS as well as double IUFD. The treatment of recurrent TTTS includes repeat laser surgery or serial amniodrainage later in gestation. Severe hemoglobin discordances can be managed by intrauterine transfusions or repeat laser coagulation. In rare cases of severe acidosis or associated anomalies, cord occlusion is needed.
- *Single IUFD* occurs in up to one-third of cases.
- The rate of *major neurologic abnormalities* after laser treatment is lower than after amniodrainage (7% vs 17%, respectively).

SELECTIVE TERMINATION OF PREGNANCY

Indications for selective feticide include serious discordant anomalies in one of the twins, severe growth restriction prior to viability, TTTS that is recurring or combined with other complications or is technically impossible to treat, and the twin reversed arterial perfusion (TRAP) sequence.

In singleton pregnancies and dichorionic twin pregnancies, feticide can easily be achieved by intracardiac or intravascular injection of potassium chloride or lidocaine. This cannot be done in MC twins, as the lethal drug may shunt from one twin to the other. More importantly, postmortem fetofetal hemorrhage is possible. Instead, surgeons can obstruct the fetal circulation directly either by endoscopic cord ligation or by a simpler endoscopic thermal coagulation. The neonatal survival rate for the healthy twin is >80%.

Procedure

- Early in gestation (as early as 16 weeks), laser energy can be used to coagulate the cord. After 20 weeks, the cord vessels become too large for laser occlusion, and the coagulation should be performed using bipolar forceps. Bipolar cord coagulation requires a 7 Fr (2.3 mm forceps) or 10 Fr (3.0 mm forceps) access to the uterus.
- A cord loop, as close as possible to the target's abdominal wall, is grabbed under ultrasound guidance and coagulated. The coagulation energy is progressively increased until a thermal effect on the cord can be visualized on ultrasound (turbu-

lence and/or steam bubbles) and arrest of flow is confirmed by Doppler studies. This is usually achieved from 25 W onwards.

- The procedure is repeated in different segments of the cord to ensure that all vessels are completely occluded.

Complications and their prevention

Early postoperative IUFD and premature rupture of membranes prior to 26 weeks can occur. The estimated learning curve is 40 procedures.

FETOSCOPIC TRACHEAL OCCLUSION FOR CONGENITAL DIAPHRAGMATIC HERNIA

Congenital diaphragmatic hernia (CDH) is a rare condition (1–2 in 5000 pregnancies). Less than half of prenatally diagnosed cases are associated with chromosomal or structural congenital anomalies (heart, central nervous system, renal, or gastrointestinal). Their prognosis is poor (<15% survival). Isolated CDH has a better prognosis, but still around 30% of fetuses will not survive. During fetal life, herniating viscera compress the developing lungs. All fetuses, therefore, have variable degrees of lung hypoplasia, which at birth may cause respiratory insufficiency.

A prenatal intervention that can trigger lung growth might improve prognosis. Open fetal surgery with anatomic repair was attempted, but was associated with a poor prognosis. Another attempt to induce lung expansion is by tracheal occlusion. This was first performed by hysterotomy – resulting in a survival rate of 33%, but with serious neurologic morbidity in the survivors.

Subsequently, a fetoscopic approach (FETO) was attempted – first by neck dissection and clipping of the trachea, and subsequently by endoluminal occlusion with an inflatable balloon. Fetal intervention does not replace postnatal therapy, but provides a better start. In the FETO Task Group, we offer prena-

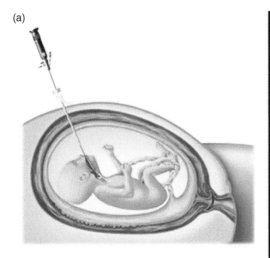

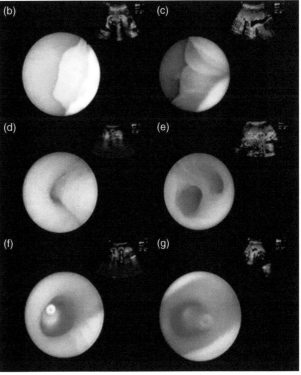

Figure 25.5 (a) Schematic drawing of percutaneous FETO. (b–g) Fetoscopic images of landmarks during percutaneous FETO: (b) epiglottis; (c) vocal cords; (d) trachea; (e) carina; (f) inflated and detached balloon; (g) vocal cords about to close over the balloon (not all images are from the same patient). (Reprinted with permission from Nelson SM, Cameron AD, Deprest JA. Fetoscopic surgery for in-utero management of congenital diaphragmatic hernia. Fetal and Maternal Medicine Review 2006; 17:69–104.)

tal surgery only to patients with *severe* isolated CDH, with no associated anomalies, liver herniation and a lung-to-head ratio (LHR) <1.0. The results of the first 20 cases were encouraging and were confirmed in a follow-up report on 28 patients. The overall survival rate in a small number of cases is about 55%, compared with a <10% survival rate in contemporary controls. The outcome of cases with extreme hypoplasia (LHR <0.6) remains poor.

Procedure

- FETO is done between 26 and 28 weeks of pregnancy. The procedure is performed under prophylactic tocolysis (atosiban and nifedipine) and antibiotics (cefazolin). Maternal analgesia is provided by combined spinal–epidural anesthesia, and the fetus is injected intramuscularly with fentanyl, pancuronium, and atropine after an adequate position for the surgery is obtained by external version.
- A 1.2 mm endoscope in a 3 mm sheath is advanced percutaneously into the fetal trachea. The landmarks are the fetal philtrum, the lips, the raphe and tongue, the epiglottis and the false and true vocal cords (Figure 25.5). A detachable balloon is positioned between the carina and vocal cords.
- Patients are admitted for 2 postoperative days and then followed by ultrasound for the position of the balloon and lung response. Removal of the balloon is carried out around 34 weeks of gestation by either fetoscopic forcipal extraction or puncture. The patient is then referred back to the referring tertiary center for planned delivery and postnatal management.

Complications and their prevention

As with other fetoscopic procedures, one of the major problems of FETO is the high rate of premature rupture of the membranes. Amniorrhexis before 28 and 32 gestational weeks occurred in 20% and 35% of cases, respectively. Experience might decrease the rate.

ACKNOWLEDGMENT

Development of instruments was supported by the European Commission, Biomed 2 Programme (EUROFOETUS) and the 5th (QLG1-CT-2002-01632) and 6th (EuroSTEC 2006-37409) framework programmes. We thank our colleagues at the Fetal Medicine Unit in Leuven (D Van Schoubroeck, R Devlieger, L Lewi, and L De Catte) and in the Eurofoetus Group (Y Ville, K Hecher, Y Dumez, U Nicolini, TH Bui, E Gratacos, and K Nicolaides) for setting up a successful consortium.

SUGGESTED READING

- Deprest J, Barki G, Lewi L, et al. Fetoscopic instrumentation and techniques. In: Van Vught J, Schulman L, eds. Fetal Medicine. New York: Marel Dekker, 2006:473–91.
- Senat MV, Deprest J, Boulvain M, et al. Endoscopic laser surgery versus serial amnioreduction for severe twin-to-twin transfusion syndrome. N Engl J Med 2004;351:136–44.
- Yamamoto M, El Murr L, Robyr R, et al. Incidence and impact of perioperative complicatons in 175 fetoscopy-guided laser coagulations of chorionic plate anastomoses in fetofetal transfusion syndrome before 26 weeks of gestation. Am J Obstet Gynecol 2005;193:1110–16.
- Lewi L, Jani J, Cannie M, et al. Intertwin anastomoses in monochorionic placentas after fetoscopic laser coagulation for twin-to-twin transfusion syndrome: Is there more than meets the eye? Am J Obstet Gynecol 2006;194:790–5.
- Lewi L, Gratacos E, Ortibus E, et al. Pregnancy and infant outcome of 80 consecutive cord coagulations in complicated monochorionic multiple pregnancies. Am J Obstet Gynecol 2006;194:782–9.
- Jani JC, Nicolaides KH, Gratacos E, Vandecruys H, Deprest JA. The Feto Task Group. Fetal lung-to-head ratio in the prediction of survival in severe left-sided diaphragmatic hernia treated by fetal endoscopic tracheal occlusion (FETO). Am J Obstet Gynecol 2006;195:1646–50.
- Deprest J, Jani J, Lewi L, et al. Fetoscopic surgery: encouraged by clinical experience and boosted by instrument innovation. Semin Fetal Neonatal Med 2006;11:398–412.

26

Basic principles of operative hysteroscopy and instrumentation

Aarathi Cholkeri-Singh and Keith B Isaacson

Pantaleoni in 1869 first performed transcervical intrauterine evaluation and treatment with hysteroscopy. He used a 12 mm cystoscope, candlelight and a concave mirror to treat polyps with silver nitrate in a 60-year-old woman. Since then, Nitze and Leiter added the optical lens to the endoscope in 1879, Heineberg used a water irrigation system in 1908, and Rubin used carbon dioxide (CO_2) in 1925. The indications to perform operative hysteroscopy include endometrial ablation and resection, myomectomy, polypectomy, tubal occlusion, metroplasty, adhesiolysis, removal of retained products of conception, visually directed biopsies of endometrial lesions, and removal of a lost intrauterine device (IUD).

A more controversial indication is endometrial resection in patients with stage 1A, grade 1 endometrial cancer. Contraindications to operative hysteroscopy include pelvic infections, excessive uterine bleeding, cervical cancer, pregnancy, and recent uterine perforation.

PREOPERATIVE PREPARATION

Before performing operative hysteroscopy, the surgeon should have a very clear preoperative plan in order to have the equipment available, as well as the ability to educate the patient on treatment options and risks of the procedure. The surgeon should use a combination of endometrial biopsy, vaginal ultrasound, sonohysterography, and/or office hysteroscopy to evaluate the endometrial cavity before performing operative

hysteroscopy. Three-dimensional ultrasound can help differentiating different types of uterine anomalies. Using images in multiple planes, the uterus could be reconstructed. Magnetic resonance imaging (MRI) is particularly useful for congenital anomalies, as well as for adenomyosis.

It is important to determine whether the patient has cervical stenosis before surgery. This could be helped by preoperative cervical softening with 200–400 µg of misoprostol or the placement of laminaria the night before surgery. The use of laminaria may be associated with overdilation and predisposes to infection. Perioperative antibiotics should be administered.

The optimal time to perform operative hysteroscopy is just after completion of menses in the early follicular phase, when the endometrium is thin. Unfortunately, abnormal bleeding, oligo-ovulation, or the surgical schedule may not permit optimal timing. This problem can be overcome by the administration of a gonadotropin-releasing hormone (GnRH) agonist 4 weeks before hysteroscopy. Besides thinning the endometrium, it decreases vascularity and fluid intravasation as well.

PROCEDURE

Anesthesia

Pain from operative hysteroscopy comes from several sources, including cervical dilatation and manipulation, uterine distention, and trauma to the endometrium and myometrium from mechanical force or heat. General or spinal anesthesia is usually used for operative hysteroscopy. Local anesthesia with intravenous sedation is reserved for those with minor intrauterine pathology that requires a short operating time. Once the patient has adequate anesthesia and is placed in the dorsal lithotomy position, a pelvic examination is performed. The bladder should be emptied with a straight red rubber or Foley catheter when a full bladder obstructs access to the cervix.

Cervical dilatation

The outer diameter of the operative hysteroscope sheath ranges from 4.5 to 10 mm (Figure 26.1). When performing operative hysteroscopy with a 4.5–5.5 mm outer diameter (OD) hysteroscope, a tenaculum may not be needed. It is needed, however, for operative hysteroscopy using a 7–10 mm OD resectoscope. If the cervix is not primed with misoprostol or laminaria, cervical dilatation is needed. This technique, while very common, may lead to cervical trauma, creation of a false passage, overdilatation, or uterine perforation.

Phillips et al described the use of dilute vasopressin injected paracervically to soften the cervix

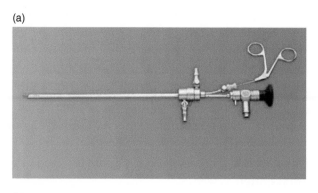

(a)

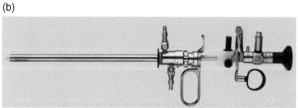

(b)

Figure 26.1 (a) 5.5 mm Betocchi operative hysteroscope. (b) 26 French Resectoscope. (Photos courtesy of Karl storz Endoscopy-America, Inc.)

before cervical dilatation. This reduces cervical trauma and decreases blood loss. The recommended dose is 0.05–0.4 U/ml, with a total dose of 4 U.

If overdilatation occurs, a removable pursestring stitch or a four-tooth tenaculum can be placed into the cervix to reduce the cervical opening and fluid leakage. Once the hysteroscope is inside the uterus, the speculum should be removed to allow full mobilization of the hysteroscope. The tenaculum on the cervix is used for gentle traction, facilitating manipulation of the hysteroscope inside the uterus.

Hysteroscope and resectoscope

Prior to utilizing the hysteroscopic equipment, it is imperative that the operating surgeon be familiar with the assembly of the resectoscope as well as with the fluid management system. The surgeon who solely relies on the ancillary staff will often find himself or herself in a difficult position when new personnel are called on to assemble and troubleshoot the hysteroscopic equipment. Continuous-flow operative hysteroscopes and resectoscopes have an inner and an outer sheath that provide channels for continuous suction and irrigation.

Light source

The most common light source is a 150–300 W halogen or xenon bulb. The hysteroscope lens is attached to a video camera to allow for visualization on a monitor. The optical lenses range from 12° to 30° angle, allowing visualization of the operative instrument as well as the intrauterine pathology.

Distending media

The uterine cavity is a potential space and has to be distended in order to operate under direct visualization. Several distending media are available:

- CO_2 gas should only be used for diagnostic hysteroscopy. Not only does it form bubbles when it comes into contact with blood, but catastrophic gas embolization has also been reported.
- High-viscosity fluid such as Dextran 70 (Hyskon) is rarely used anymore. Its use is associated with hypertonicity, allergy reactions, and a tendency to cause sticking of the hysteroscopic equipment.

- Low-viscosity fluids either contain physiologic levels of electrolytes (saline or Lactated Ringer's solution) or are electrolyte-free (1.5% glycine, 3% sorbitol, and 5% mannitol). Cold scissors, lasers, or bipolar instruments can be used with electrolyte-containing distention medium. However, it disperses electrical current. Accordingly, when using monopolar energy, electrolyte-free solutions should be utilized.

Accessory instruments

Accessory mechanical instruments for operative hysteroscope can be rigid, semirigid, or flexible. The tips are sharp- or blunt-tipped scissors, grasping forceps, or biopsy forceps. The rigid instruments are fixed permanently to the end of the sheath, enabling the physician to move the scope and instrument as one unit. Simple operative procedures such as removal of small endometrial and endocervical polyps, directed biopsy, and lysis of adhesions can be done with semirigid graspers, biopsy forceps, or scissors placed through a 4.5–5.5 mm OD continuous-flow hysteroscope (Figure 26.2).

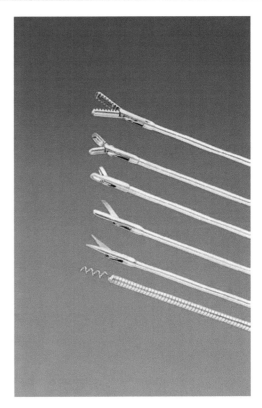

Figure 26.2 Various Semirigid Instrument Tips. (Photo courtesy of Karl Storz Endoscopy-America, Inc.)

Tissue removal

The availability of hysteroscopic morcellators enables simultaneous resection and removal of submucous myomas and polyps (Figure 26.3). Removal of larger lesions requires a resectoscope of outer diameter 7–10 mm. The electrode can be a cutting loop, a roller ball or barrel, a vaporizing electrode, or a spiked cutting tip (Figure 26.4). The loop electrode is used for removal of submucosal myomas or polyps, metroplasty, or endometrial resection.

Newly available is the Chip-E-Vac radiofrequency system (Richard Wolf Medical Instruments Corporation, Vernon Hills, IL), which contains a loop electrode and simultaneously removes tissue chips while resecting (Figure 26.5). The cutting tips, such as the bipolar twizzle tips, are used for septum resection and bisection of large lesions.

Electrodes

The roller ball or barrel is mainly for endometrial ablation (Figure 26.6). Endometrial ablation can be performed with equivalent results using 50–100 W of either a pure coagulating or cutting current. When cutting intrauterine lesions, we use 50–100 W of pure cutting current. Vaporizing electrodes operate at a higher power density, vaporizing the tissue. These electrodes do not provide tissue for pathology and they create bubbles, which impairs visualization. Lasers can also be used for operative hysteroscopes. However, due to their expense and the availability of cheaper modalities, hysteroscopic lasers are rarely used today.

Post procedure

Patients are usually discharged a few hours following the procedure. Minimal to moderate cramping is relieved with nonsteroidal anti-inflammatory drugs. Most anesthesiologists will administer ketorolac postoperatively to minimize uterine cramping. Some patients will experience mild to heavy spotting, which usually resolves within 24–72 hours.

Patients can resume normal daily activities within 24–72 hours. We advise them not to insert anything

(a)

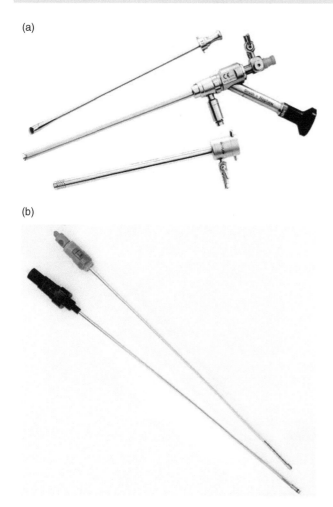

(b)

Figure 26.3 (a) Smith & Nephew, Inc. hysteroscope. (b) Smith & Nephew, Inc morcellator accessory instruments. (Photos courtesy of Smith & Nephew, Inc.)

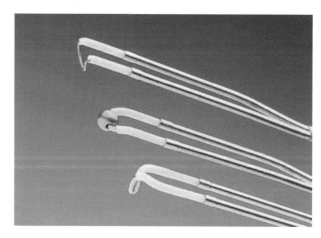

Figure 26.4 Operative resectoscope accesory RF electrodes. (Photos courtesy of Karl Storz Endoscopy-America, Inc.)

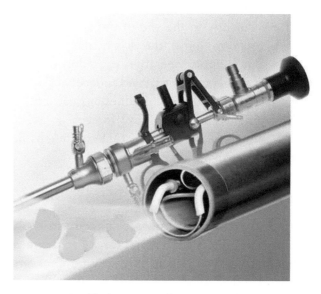

Figure 26.5 Wolf Chip E-Vac illustration. (Photo courtesy of Richard Wolf Medical Instruments Corp.)

into the vagina for 2 weeks. This is to decrease the risk of infection.

COMPLICATIONS AND THEIR PREVENTION

- Infection related to the procedure is rare. Prophylactic antibiotics are not usually recommended.
- Bleeding can occur either from cervical lacerations or from the uterine cavity during the procedure. Cervical lacerations are managed with simple interrupted sutures. When the bleeding is from the uterine cavity, bimanual compression is the first step to decrease the bleeding. If this fails, a 30 cm² Foley balloon is placed into the

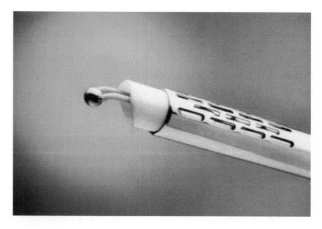

Figure 26.6 Resectoscope Tip with Rollerball electrode. (Photo courtesy of Karl Storz Endoscopy-America, Inc.)

uterine cavity and inflated with 15–30 cm^2 of saline. The Foley catheter can be removed in 4–24 hours. In the rare situation when the bleeding persists, one could consider uterine artery embolization.

- Uterine perforation can occur with blind instrumentation such as cervical dilators. If perforation occurs with an active electrode, laparoscopy or exploratory laparotomy should be performed to rule out visceral and/or vascular injury. If no injuries are identified, the patient must be followed for signs and symptoms of infection, bowel perforation, or bleeding. The possibility of uterine perforation using an active electrode can be reduced by retracting the electrode toward the surgeon.

- Intravasation of fluid from distention media can occur through open venous channels in the uterus:
  - High-viscosity fluid, such as Hyskon, is hyperosmotic and has been associated with pulmonary edema and coagulopathies at deficit volumes of 350 cm^3. Anaphylactic reactions have been reported.
  - Low-viscosity electrolyte solutions are isotonic. They can cause fluid overload and pulmonary edema. If the deficit is over 1 liter, a diuretic such as 10 mg of furosemide should be administered intravenously. A Foley catheter is inserted into the bladder for measurement of urinary output.
  - Low-viscosity electrolyte-free solutions are hypotonic, and can cause water intoxication and hyponatremia. Symptoms of mild hyponatremia are nonspecific, and include postoperative nausea, vomiting and irritability at serum sodium levels of 130–135 mEq/l (Chapter 36). With severe hyponatremia, patient can develop hypotension, bradycardia, convulsions, brainstem herniation, and death. We recommend the use of a fluid monitoring system.

CONCLUSION

It is beyond the scope of this chapter to provide detail instruction on all the hysteroscopic procedures that can be performed with the operative hysteroscope. Given this, there are basic principles that should be followed that apply to all operative hysteroscopic procedures. Listed below are examples of such principles, not in order of importance:

- Preoperative planning – as previously stated, the uterine cavity should be assessed prior to the operative procedure to eliminate the possibility of unexpected pathology, which may alter appropriate patient management.

- Consider cervical softening agents, such as misoprostol, laminaria, or dilute vasopressin solution, to reduce the risks of cervical trauma and uterine perforation.

- Establish a fluid management protocol within the hospital that is agreed upon by the nursing staff, anesthesiologists, and the operating surgeons. This reduces the risks of conflict as the fluid deficit approaches patient safety limits.

- Only use physiologic distention media unless monopolar energy is necessary for resection or ablation.

- Attempt to avoid cutting myometrium whenever possible. When removing type I and type II myomas hysteroscopically, the pseudocapsule should be identified and the loop electrode should always stay in this plane or within the myoma. This technique will minimize the risk of uterine perforation.

- Use the minimal intrauterine distention pressure that will allow for adequate flow of media and surgeon visibility. The lower the pressure, the lower amount of fluid intravasation and the more intramural component of a myoma will protrude within the uterine cavity. It is acceptable to go above the mean arterial pressure if necessary for good visualization. However, the surgeon should terminate the procedure when the maximum fluid deficit is reached.

- Most bleeding is due to venous leakage. This will stop spontaneously and does not require electorsurgical dessication

SUGGESTED READING

- Phillips DR, Nathanson HG, Milim SJ, et al. The effect of dilute vasopressin solution on the force needed for cervical dilatation: a randominzed controlled trial. Obstet Gynecol 1997; 89(4):507–11.

- Taskin O, Yalcinoglu A, Kucuk S, et al. The degree of fluid absorption during hysteroscopic surgery in patients pretreated with goserelin. J Am Asssoc Gynecol Laparosc 1996;3(4):555-9

- Cohen S. Operative Laparoscopy & Hysteroscopy. New York: Churchill Livingstone Inc, 1996:227–302.

- Valle RF. Manual of Clinical Hysteroscopy. United Kingdom: Taylor & Francis, 2005:1–160.

- Baggish Ms, Barbot J, Valle RF. Diagnostic and Operative Hyseroscopy: A Text and Atlas. Chicago: Year Book Medical Publishers, Inc. 1989:50–185.

27

Office hysteroscopy

Stefano Bettocchi, Oronzo Ceci, Giovanni Pontrelli, Tatjana Dosev, Anna Franca Laera, Clementina Cantatore, and Luigi Selvaggi

Hysteroscopy can be performed in an office setting (*outpatient hysteroscopy*) or as a day-case procedure, under general anaesthesia (*inpatient hysteroscopy*). The advantages of office hysteroscopy are reduced anaesthetic risk, reduced time and cost of the procedure, and patient preference compared with inpatient hysteroscopy. Office hysteroscopy may be indicated in any situation in which a major or minor intrauterine or cervical anomaly is suspected and for the purpose of endometrial surveillance during hormonal treatment.

Instead of inpatient hysteroscopy, outpatient hysteroscopy might be offered to patients who not wish or cannot undergo general or local anaesthesia and to virgin patients who wish to preserve the integrity of their hymen (vaginoscopic approach).

INSTRUMENTATION

Rigid hysteroscope

The availability of hysteroscopes with a diameter of 1.2–3 mm and a working channel of <5 mm has allowed physicians to perform directed biopsy and to treat minor intrauterine pathologies. One of the newest hysteroscopes is the Office Continuous Flow Operative Hysteroscope Size 4 (Karl Storz, Tuttlingen, Germany), with a 2.0 mm rod–lens system, 30° fore–oblique view, and an outer diameter of 4.0 mm. It has two sheaths (one for irrigation and one for suction), an operative 5 Fr canal (approximately 1.6 mm), and is oval in shape – ideal for atraumatic insertion of the scope into the cervix. In addition, it has a high visual quality, brightness, angle of view, and a field of view comparable to that of a standard 4.0 mm telescope.

Distention of the uterus is obtained using an electronic suction–irrigation pump (Endomat, Karl Storz) that can maintain a constant intrauterine pressure around 30/40 mmHg, necessary to avoid overdistention of the uterus and reduce patient discomfort. A high-intensity xenon or halogen light of at least 250 W is necessary for the best visualization.

In the last few years, smaller-diameter flexible hysteroscopes have demonstrated in several studies some advantages in term of patient discomfort compared with standard rigid ones. Disadvantages are a higher cost of equipment purchase and maintenance, difficulties in cleaning, disinfection, and sterilization, greater fragility, standard 0° angle of vision, and reduced image size on the monitor compared with the standard hysteroscopy.

Flexible hysteroscope

Recent improvements in fiberoptic technology have allowed the realization of a semirigid 3.2 mm mini-hysteroscope (Versascope, Gynecare, Ethicon, Inc., Sommerville, NJ). Compared with a standard hysteroscope, it is associated with less trauma and is easy to use. However, it cannot match the image quality of rod–lens-based telescope systems. Visualization of the uterine cavity with the flat tip of the scope with standard 0° angle of vision may also be impaired.

Distention media

Carbon dioxide gas

Office hysteroscopy can be done using CO_2 gas as distending medium. However, CO_2 tends to produce gas bubbles, especially when it mixes with blood; obscuring vision. These bubbles can be confused with intrauterine adhesions or synechiae. Some soft and small intrauterine pathology can be missed when using the CO_2, due to compression of the gas on the tissues.

Normal saline

Compared with CO_2, the use of normal saline is associated with less patient discomfort, is more cost-effective, and provides better vision in the case of intrauterine bleeding. In any event, blood and mucus should be carefully removed from the cervical opening with a dry swab. For office operative hysteroscopy, we use normal saline as distending medium. We recommend the use of a continuous-flow system together with an electronic suction– irrigation device. This provides clear vision in the case of bleeding or the presence of thick mucus.

Versapoint system

This system (Gynecare, Ethicon, Inc.) consists of a high-frequency bipolar electrosurgical generator and coaxial bipolar electrodes designed to cut, desiccate (coagulate), and vaporize tissue. The 1.6mm-diameter (5 Fr), 36 cm-long, flexible bipolar electrode can be used through any operating hysteroscope. Each bipolar electrode consists of an active electrode located at the tip and a return electrode located on the shaft, separated by a ceramic insert. The possibility of using a bipolar electrode allows hysteroscopy to be performed using normal saline solution.

This system avoids both stray electrical energy and the risks of nonelectrolyte distending medium. Because it vaporizes tissue, the procedure can be accomplished more quickly, as vision is not obscured by chips. More precise vaporization also avoids cutting into myometrium. There are three types of electrodes: the twizzle, specifically for precise and controlled vaporization (resembling cutting); the spring, used for diffuse tissue vaporization; and the ball, to coagulate tissues. The twizzle electrode is preferred to the others because is a more precise 'cutting' instrument and can work closer to the myometrium with lower power setting and consequently with less patient discomfort.

The generator provides different modes of operation (waveform): the vapor cut waveform, resembling a cut mode (the acronyms are VC1, VC2, and VC3, where VC3 corresponds to the mildest energy flowing into the tissue), the blend waveform (BL1 and BL2), and the desiccation waveform, resembling a coagulation mode (DES). The generator is connected to the 5 Fr electrode via a flexible cable. Once connected, the generator automatically adjusts to the default setting (VC1 and 100 W).

The Versapoint system has been used to treat a variety of intrauterine lesions with the administration of conscious sedation, with or without paracervical block, with the use of general anaesthesia, and recently without any analgesia or anaesthesia.

VAGINOSCOPIC APPROACH

We have used this technique to decrease patient discomfort without the use of a speculum or tenaculum. This approach is ideal for office hysteroscopy in women with stenotic vagina or in virgins.

The vagina is first distended with the saline solution and the hysteroscope is inserted into the vagina to visualize the cervical opening (Figures 27.1 and 27.2). Subsequently, the operator introduces the

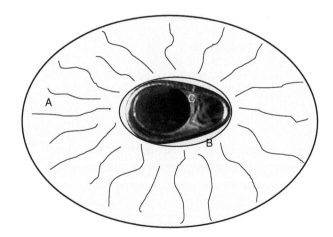

Figure 27.1 View of the internal cervical opening and the hysteroscope profile in a traditional introduction: A, cervix; B, internal cervical os; C, hysteroscope profile.

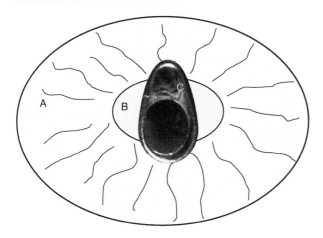

Figure 27.2 View of the internal cervical opening and hysteroscope profile after 90° rotation: A, cervix; B, internal cervical os; C, hysteroscope profile.

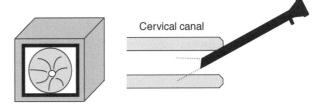

Figure 27.3 Wrong view on the screen corresponding to inappropriate alignment of the instrument with the cervical canal.

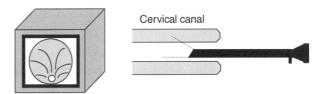

Figure 27.4 Correct view on the screen corresponding to appropriate alignment of the instrument with the cervical canal.

hysteroscope into the cervical canal and then the uterine cavity. Correct insertion can be assisted manually with the operator's hands.

The fore-oblique view of 12° or 30° is useful to examine the uterine cavity, but can complicate the introduction of the scope into the cervical canal. The image localized in the middle of the screen is in fact located 12° or 30° lower. On the monitor, the image of the cervical canal should appear in the lower half of the screen and not in its center (Figures 27.3 and 27.4).

DIAGNOSTIC HYSTEROSCOPY

Hysteroscopy must be performed in the early proliferative phase of the cycle when the endometrium is thin, usually flat and hypotrophic, similar to the appearance of the endometrium of a postmenopausal woman (Figure 27.5). By placing the hysteroscope close to the endometrium, one can see the vascular pattern, gland openings, and pathologic features such as endometrial hyperplasia and endometrial cancer.

The hysteroscopic appearance of endometrial hyperplasia is variable and sometimes it is very difficult to distinguish it from secretory endometrium. Simple hyperplasia is characterized by a thick endometrium, sometimes with a polypoid aspect; glandular ostium appears dilated and yellowish in color. Atypical hyperplasia is characterized by hemorrhagic, necrotic areas and gross proliferations that could distort the entire uterine cavity. Endometrial

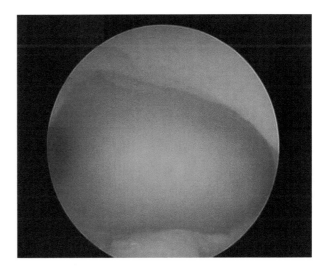

Figure 27.5 Normal cavity.

vessels appear irregular in shape and branching. The hysteroscopic appearance of atypical hyperplasia could generate problems in differential diagnosis with endometrial carcinoma, so histologic confirmation is mandatory.

TARGETED HYSTEROSCOPIC BIOPSY

Instead of a punch biopsy, we propose a grasp biopsy to collect sufficient endometrium for histologic examination. The biopsy forceps are placed, with jaws open, in contact with the endometrium; they are then pushed into the tissue for about 0.5–1 cm. Once a large portion of mucosa has been detached, the jaws are closed and then the whole hysteroscope is pulled out of the uterine cavity, without pulling the tip of the instrument back into the channel.

OFFICE OPERATIVE HYSTEROSCOPY

With the development of smaller-diameter scopes with working channels and continuous-flow systems, it is now possible to treat several uterine, cervical, and vaginal pathologies in an office setting without cervical dilatation and consequently without anaesthesia or analgesia.

Mechanical operative instruments (scissors, biopsy cup, grasper, and corkscrew) were for a long time the only way to apply the 'see-and-treat' procedure in the office setting. The advent of bipolar technology, with introduction of several types of 5 Fr electrodes, has increased the number of pathologies that can be created in this way, with the resectoscope and operating room being reserved for a few cases.

Polypectomy (Figure 27.6)

Small polyps (<0.5 cm) can be removed using hysteroscopic scissors and/or crocodile forceps. Cervical polyps have to be treated with scissors because their fibrotic base precludes the use of grasping forceps. For endometrial polyps, the technique is

to grasp the base with open jaws, close the instrument, and push it gently toward the uterine fundus. The procedure has to be repeated several times until the polyp is detached.

A large polyp can be removed intact, with the Versapoint twizzle electrode, only if the opening of the internal cervical is sufficiently wide for its extraction. Otherwise, it must be sliced from its free edge to the base into two or three fragments, small enough to be pulled out through the uterine cavity using 5 Fr grasping forceps with teeth. To remove the entire base of the polyp without going too deeply into the myometrium, in some cases the twizzle electrode is bent by 25°–30°, enough to obtain the shape of hook electrode.

Myomectomy (Figure 27.7)

The size limit for an office hysteroscopic myomectomy is 1.5–2 cm. We use a technique similar to that of polypectomy. However, due its firmness, a myoma has to be divided into two half-spheres, each of which is sliced and removed with grasping forceps. The intramural part of the myoma is first separated from the capsule using mechanical instruments (grasping forceps or scissors). Once the intramural section becomes submucosal, it is treated in the same fashion.

Uterine septum and synechiae (Figures 27.8 and 27.9)

Uterine septum or intrauterine synechiae can be cut using scissors or bipolar electrodes. Because hystero-

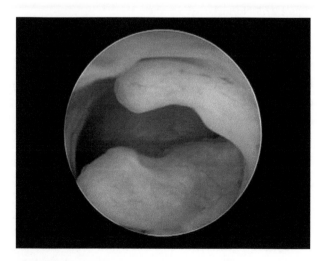

Figure 27.6 Endometrial polyp.

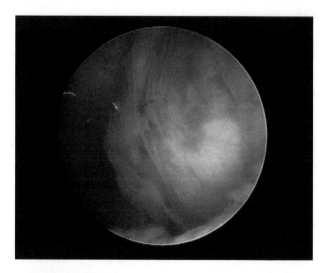

Figure 27.7 Submucous myoma.

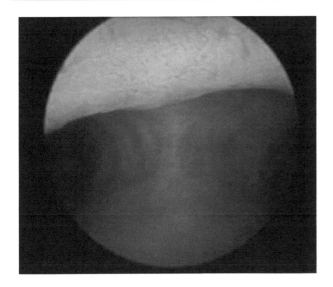

Figure 27.8 Uterine septum.

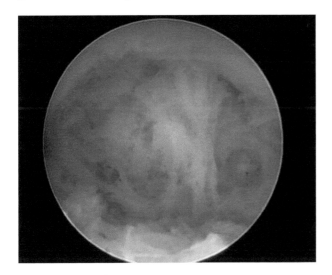

Figure 27.9 Synechiae.

scopic visualization cannot differentiate a bicornuate uterus from a septate uterus, we undertake magnetic resonance imaging (MRI) before surgery or perform a combined hysteroscopy and laparoscopy.

The septum is progressively divided, starting from the proximal part, equidistantly from the anterior and posterior uterine walls. The decision to stop incision of the septum is taken when significant bleeding is observed, as well as pinkish tissue. We believe that office hysteroscopic metroplasty without local anesthesia is particularly helpful. The patient will experience pain when the muscular tissue is reached. At that instant, the metroplasty must be stopped – regardless of the length of the septum left. This allows preservation of the myometrium from unnecessary damage.

Tubal sterilization

Hysteroscopic tubal sterilization using Essure (Conceptus, Incorporated, Mountain View, CA), can also be performed in an office setting. The device is a titanium stainless steel and nickel expanding-spring device (2 mm in diameter and 4 cm long), which contains Dacron fibres that induce an inflammatory reaction and a subsequent fibrosis of the intramural tubal lumen. The device is inserted into the tubal ostium under hysteroscopic vision.

SUGGESTED READING

- Kremer C, Duffy S, Moroney M. Patient satisfaction with outpatient hysteroscopy versus day case hysteroscopy: randomised controlled trial. BMJ 2000;320: 279–82.
- Cicinelli E, Parisi C, Galantino P, et al. Reliability, feasibility, and safety of minihysteroscopy with a vaginoscopic approach: experience with 6,000 cases. Fertil Steril 2003;80:199–202.
- De Angelis C, Santoro G, Re ME, et al. Office hysteroscopy and compliance: mini-hysteroscopy versus traditional hysteroscopy in a randomized trial. Hum Reprod 2003;18:2441–5.
- Bettocchi S, Selvaggi L. A vaginoscopic approach to reduce the pain of office hysteroscopy. J Am Assoc Gynecol Laparosc 1997;4:255–8.
- Bettocchi S, Ceci O, Di Venere R, et al. Advanced operative office hysteroscopy without anaesthesia: analysis of 501 cases treated with a 5 Fr bipolar electrode. Hum Reprod 2002;17:2435–8.
- Bettocchi S, Ceci O, Nappi L, et al. Operative office hysteroscopy without anesthesia: analysis of 4863 cases performed with mechanical instruments. J Am Assoc Gynecol Laparosc 2004;11:59–61.

28

Flexible hysteroscopy

Amudha Thangavelu and Sean Duffy

In comparison with rigid hysteroscopy, flexible hysteroscopy is associated with less discomfort, allows for easy passage of the endocervical canal, enables easy maneuvering around submucous fibroids or endometrial polyps, and in some cases obviates the need for cervical dilatation. It is a safe, successful, well-tolerated, and acceptable procedure when performed in the outpatient setting. Indications and contraindications of flexible hysteroscopy are similar to those of conventional hysteroscopy.

EQUIPMENT

Most flexible hysteroscopes (Figure 28.1) are about 3 mm in diameter and consist of:

- a proximal extremity that holds the ocular system with the focus ring, a distal manipulator, opening to the operating channel, and an exit site for the operating sheath
- a flexible main sheath that carries the fiberoptic bundles from the light, the operating channel, and the bundles that carry the reflected image to the eyepiece
- a distal extremity that is flexible and provides a 100° bidirectional field of view
- a light connection

An excellent light source is required in order to enable good visualization of the endometrial cavity. A video system is normally used in order to obtain hard-copy images and also to enable the patient to observe the findings. The distending medium can be either carbon dioxide (CO_2) gas or normal saline.

SETTING

An appropriate setting is important to ensure the success of an outpatient hysteroscopy. A good-sized room with adequate privacy and changing facilities should be available, with a separate area for consultation if the patient wishes to discuss any concerns. A reclining chair that can be electrically tilted to the required position is preferred (Figure 28.2). It is important to have at least two nurses in the

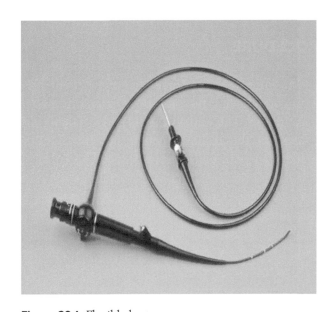

Figure 28.1 Flexible hysteroscope.

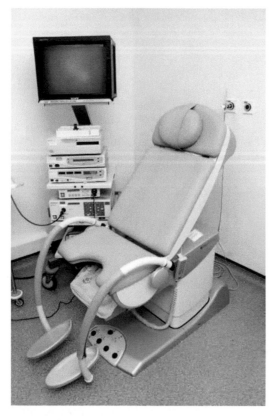

Figure 28.2 Reclining electrically operated chair and hysteroscopy stack.

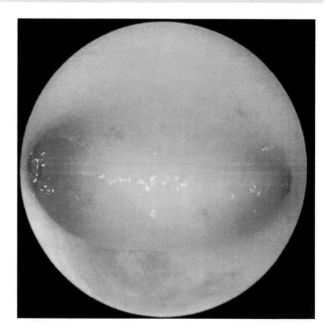

Figure 28.3 Normal endometrial cavity.

clinic – one to assist the operator in clinic while the other can reassure the patient and act as a chaperone.

PROCEDURE

• The importance of counselling the patient prior to commencing the procedure cannot be under-estimated. The patient should be made comfort-able on the reclining couch and tilted to the required position. After inspecting the vulva for any abnormalities, a bimanual examination must be performed in order to determine if the uterus is anteverted or retroverted. A Cuscoe's speculum is inserted to visualize the cervix. Most patients do not require any analgesia for flexible hysteroscopy. If cervical dilatation is necessary, a tenaculum or vulsellum may be used to straighten the cervical canal, and the internal os is dilated using graded Hegar dilators.

• The hysteroscope is introduced into the cervical canal under direct vision and advanced slowly, following the contour of the endocervical canal. Once inside the endometrial cavity, a panoramic view should be obtained, which helps to map the location of abnormalities (Figure 28.3). The length of the uterine cavity should be noted with the tip of the scope at the fundus. It is important to examine the fundus, uterine cornua, and the anterior and posterior walls carefully. If possible, a still or video image of these and any other abnor-malities should be obtained for documentation. The hysteroscope is then gradually withdrawn under direct vision to examine the endocervical canal again.

• A directed endometrial biopsy or removal of small polyps (Figure 28.4) may be undertaken at the time of hysteroscopy using a snare, biopsy forceps, or grasping forceps. If a directed biopsy is not required, a Pipelle endometrial sampler may be used to obtain tissue for histopathologic eval-uation.

Hysteroscopy is considered failed when access to the uterine cavity cannot be obtained or when the view is suboptimal. Failure to gain access to the uterine cavity may be due to cervical stenosis or pain. The view is

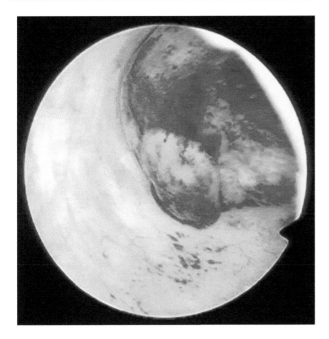

Figure 28.4 Endometrial polyp.

considered to be suboptimal when blood, debris, or bubbles prevent the operator from examining the entire uterine cavity, tubal ostia, or cervical canal. In the event of a failed hysteroscopy, an inpatient hysteroscopy should be arranged.

We recommend documentation of the procedure, including photography. This should involve a complete history, including the indication for the hysteroscopy. The size and type of the scope, the distention medium, and the use of anesthesia, tenaculum, or dilators should be recorded. The findings should be documented in a systematic manner, and should include the appearance of the vulva, vagina, ectocervix, endocervical canal, and endometrial cavity.

Any complications that occur during the procedure should be noted. Finally, it is important to record any discussion with the patient, and a management plan should be outlined.

COMPLICATIONS AND THEIR PREVENTION

Complications are rare and usually minor.

- Pain is the most common complication, and may occasionally result in the procedure being abandoned.
- Vasovagal reaction may occur in some patients – usually secondary to cervical dilatation.
- Infection is a rare complication. Routine use of antibiotics is not usually recommended.
- Trauma to the genital tract (false passage or uterine perforation) is rare, but may occur during cervical dilatation.

SUGGESTED READING

- Marsh F, Duffy S. The technique and overview of flexible hysteroscopy. Obstet Gynecol Clin North Am 2004;31:655–68.
- Kremer C, Barik S, Duffy S. Flexible outpatient hysteroscopy without anaesthesia: a safe, successful and well tolerated procedure. Br J Obstet Gynaecol 1998;105:672–6.
- Trew GH. Hysteroscopy and hysteroscopic surgery. Curr Obstet Gynaecol 2004;14:183–90.
- Baxter A, Beck B, Phillips, K. A randomised controlled trial of rigid and flexible hysteroscopy in an outpatient setting. Gynaecol Endosc 2002; 11:229–35.

29

Hysteroscopic treatment of intrauterine adhesions

Alaa El-Ghobashy, Geoffrey Trew, and Peter O'Donovan

Asherman described two different types of traumatic synechiae: stenosis or obliteration of the cervical canal in the vicinity of the internal os, and partial or complete obliteration of the uterine cavity by conglutination of the opposing walls. Dilatation and curettage immediately after a delivery or a miscarriage is the main cause of intrauterine adhesions (75%). Infection might contribute to the development of intrauterine synechiae in 26% of cases. Other causes are cesarean or uterine surgery unassociated with pregnancy. The overall pregnancy rate after hysteroscopic adhesiolysis is 43%, with a live birth rate of 32%.

The most severe form of intrauterine synechiae is related to endometrial tuberculosis, where the entire endometrial cavity may be completely lost, including the cornual regions. Its prognosis is poor.

DIAGNOSIS

- Amenorrhea in the presence of ovulation suggests target organ defect such as intrauterine synechiae.
- Sonohysterography and hysterosalpingography (HSG; Figure 29.1) may show complete or partial obliteration of the uterine cavity. HSG is generally more sensitive and specific, especially if the adhesions are thin or not calcified.
- Diagnostic hysteroscopy allows accurate evaluation of the uterine cavity (Figures 29.2–29.4).
- Classification of intrauterine adhesions is critical, as it affects treatment outcome. The scoring system in the American Fertility Society classification incorporates the extent of the uterine cavity

involvement (score 1: less than one-third; 2: one-third or two-thirds; 4: over two-thirds), the type of adhesions (score 1: filmy; 2: filmy and dense; 4: dense) and menstruation (score 0: normal; 2: hypomenorrhea; 4: amenorrhea). Scores of 1–4 indicate mild cases, scores of 5–8 indicate moderate cases, and scores of 9–12 indicate severe cases with poor outcome.

PROCEDURE

- Hysteroscopic resection of intrauterine adhesions is a safe and effective procedure for restoring normal menstruation. This could be aided with the use of laparoscopy. The resulting carbon dioxide pneumoperitoneum separates the uterus from the surrounding organs in the event of

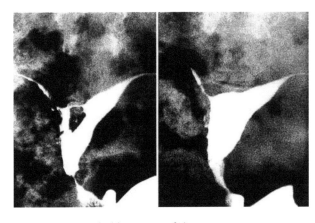

Figure 29.1 Partial obliteration of the uterine cavity.

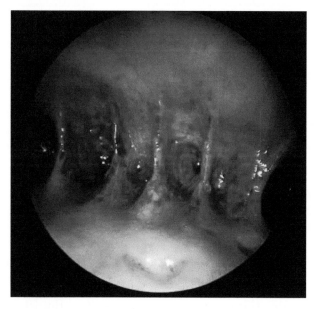

Figure 29.2 Thick intrauterine adhesion involving one-third of the uterine cavity.

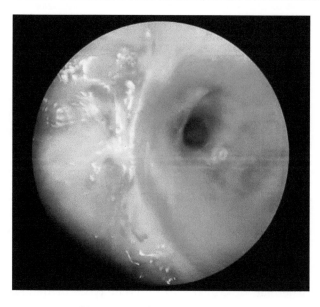

Figure 29.4 Obliteration of over two-thirds of the uterine cavity.

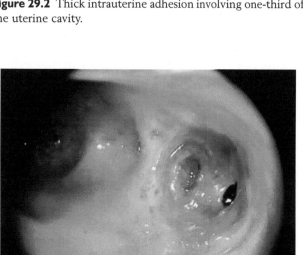

Figure 29.3 Dense intrauterine adhesions.

uterine perforation. Transillumination of the myometrium allows safe dissection and limits unnecessary surgical intervention. Knowledge of the presence of the cornual cavity allows the surgeon to create a passage between the internal cervical os and the cornual areas, and thus be able to fashion a 'septum-like' structure from the intrauterine adhesions. The adhesions can then be divided, and subsequently the bases will retract. We use prophylactic intraoperative antibiotics.

- The cervix is dilated to Hegar 10 to allow the passage of a 10 mm rigid operative hysteroscope. Smaller operative hysteroscopes can also be used in some patients. We use hysteroscopic scissors to cut the adhesions (Figure 29.5). The distention medium is usually normal saline. Utilization of an electrosurgical device such as a knife or monopolar needle (Figure 29.6) necessitates the use of glycine 1.5% as distending medium. A cutting current (40–50 W) should be used because of its safety in comparison with a coagulating current.

- Release of adhesions starts just above the internal cervical os and progresses upward toward the uterine fundus. Filmy adhesions should be separated first, followed by fibrous/tough ones. Ball diathermy can be used to control bleeding points resulting from dissection. This technique should be employed sparingly, however, as it can in itself be adhesiogenic.

- If the cavity is blocked at the level of the cervical canal, we use a fine silver probe to dilate the cervix under abdominal ultrasound guidance. Direct real-time ultrasound control can be used with the probe to break down cervical adhesions and allow the probe to be accurately directed to pockets of endometrium seen sonographically. This creates a channel, into which the hysteroscope can be inserted and further adhesiolysis performed.

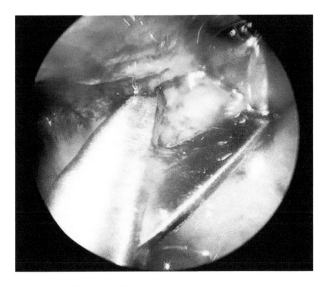

Figure 29.5 Cutting adhesions using hysteroscopic scissors.

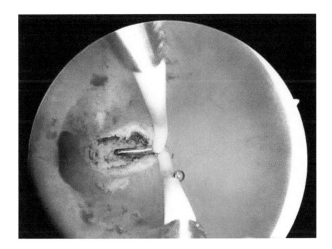

Figure 29.6 Cutting adhesions with a monopolar needle.

- Other methods have been used to manage intrauterine adhesions, including the Versapoint device (Gynecare, Ethicon, Inc., Sommerville, NJ), the neodymium : yttrium aluminum garnet (Nd:YAG) laser, and mechanical disruption using pressure lavage under ultrasound guidance (PLUG). This last technique allows lysis of mild filmy intrauterine adhesions. However, its efficacy in moderate and its application to severe adhesions are limited.
- A plastic intrauterine contraceptive device can be left in place for up to 4 weeks to act as a

splint to prevent apposition of the uterine walls. It can also perform adhesiolysis of de novo adhesions on removal. The patient is advised to use conjugated estrogen (1.25–2.5 mg daily) for 2 months, together with progesterone in the last week of the cycle to help stimulate growth of the endometrium.

- In the past, we inserted a Foley catheter balloon filled with 5–10 ml fluid into the uterine cavity for 10–15 days to prevent adhesions. This procedure has many disadvantages, including hospitalization for 2 weeks, infection, pain, and cervical incompetence. The balloon might also impede normal growth of the endometrium by pressing on the uterine wall. We no longer recommend its use.
- Acunzo et al reported that the intrauterine application of autocrosslinked hyaluronic acid (ACP) gel following hysteroscopic adhesiolysis significantly reduces the incidence of postoperative formation of intrauterine adhesions. In addition, it reduced the severity of these adhesions.
- The use of a fresh amnion graft over the inflated balloon of a Foley catheter for 2 weeks has also been advocated.

COMPLICATIONS AND THEIR PREVENTION

- Besides complications related to hysteroscopy in general, lysis of intrauterine adhesions carries a specific risk of uterine perforation. Attention should be paid to lateral adhesions, where uterine perforation is likely to occur if aggressive adhesiolysis is attempted. Performing the procedure under ultrasound guidance or laparoscopic control is beneficial.
- Recurrence of intrauterine adhesions and restoration of menstruation are case-dependent. The success rate can be increased with the use of intrauterine devices and estrogen postoperatively.
- Pregnancy after lysis of intrauterine adhesion is associated with an increased risk of miscarriage and hemorrhage because of abnormal placentation. The patient should also be warned of the possibility of placenta accreta.

SUGGESTED READING

- Asherman JG. [Intrauterine adhesions.] Bull Fed Soc Gynecol Obstet Lang Fr 1952;4:807–14.
- Friedler S, Margalioth EJ, Kafka I, Yaffe H. Incidence of post-abortion intra-uterine adhesions evaluated by hysteroscopy – a prospective study. Hum Reprod 1993;8:442–4.
- American Fertility Society. The American Fertility Society classifications of adnexal adhesions, distal tubal occlusion, tubal occlusion secondary to tubal ligation, tubal pregnancies, mullerian anomalies and intrauterine adhesions. Fertil Steril 1988;49: 944–55.
- Coccia ME, Becattini C, Bracco GL, et al. Pressure lavage under ultrasound guidance: a new approach for outpatient treatment of intrauterine adhesions. Fertil Steril 2001;75:601–6.
- Acunzo G, Guida M, Pellicano M, et al. Effectiveness of auto-cross-linked hyaluronic acid gel in the prevention of intrauterine adhesions after hysteroscopic adhesiolysis: a prospective, randomized, controlled study. Hum Reprod 2003;18:1918–21.
- Amer MI, Abd-El-Maeboud KH. Amnion graft following hysteroscopic lysis of intrauterine adhesions. J Obstet Gynaecol Res 2006;32:559–66.

30

Hysteroscopic polypectomy and myomectomy

Alaa El-Ghobashy and Peter O'Donovan

The most common intrauterine lesions causing excessive uterine bleeding are endometrial polyps and submucous fibroid. An endometrial polyp is a localized overgrowth of endometrial tissue covered by epithelium, and contains variable amounts of glands, stroma, and blood vessels, forming a projection above the endometrial surface (Figures 30.1 and 30.2). The prevalence of endometrial polyps in women with abnormal uterine bleeding is 10–20%. Polyps might be sessile or pedunculated, and rarely include foci of neoplastic growth.

Uterine fibroids (leiomyomas) are the most common benign neoplasms in women of reproductive age. They represent abnormal growth of uterine smooth muscle cells, with limited malignant transformation (<1%). One study showed that over 25% of women report clinical symptoms caused by fibroids.

Investigations of intrauterine lesions include transvaginal ultrasonography and hysterosonography, with hysteroscopy as the gold standard. Hysteroscopy allows panoramic inspection of the uterine cavity and direct biopsy of the lesions.

Diagnostic hysteroscopy is best performed in the early proliferative phase of the menstrual cycle. Thin endometrium facilitates visualization of the uterine cavity. Alternatively, one dose of a long-acting gonadotropin-releasing hormone analog (GnRHa) such as leuprolide acetate 3.75 mg intramuscularly can be administered 4 weeks before hysteroscopy to remove the lesion.

The surgeon should classify uterine fibroids prior to surgery. The European Society of Gynaecological Endoscopy classifies submucous fibroids into type 0 (completely intracavitary: Figure 30.3), type 1 (intramural extension <50%: Figure 30.4), and type 2 (intramural extension >50%: Figure 30.5). Traditionally, uterine polyps are removed by curettage. However, this is an outdated and blind procedure. More importantly, it misses a quarter of endometrial and 10% of intrauterine polyps.

PROCEDURES

Hysteroscopic polypectomy

Hysteroscopic polypectomy allows complete removal of polyps under direct vision. The operative procedure is performed using a resectoscope with either a 7 or a 9 mm outer operative sheath. General or spinal anesthesia can be used to facilitate dilatation of the cervical canal. The resectoscope is inserted into the uterine cavity and sterile 1.5% glycine solution is used for uterine distention and irrigation. Fluid infusion should be controlled either with a Hamou Hysteromat (Karl Storz, Tuttlinge, Germany) or by strictly recording the infused and drained fluid from the continuous-flow hysteroscope. Alternatively, hydrostatic pressure can be used to provide positive pressure by hanging the glycine bag 90–100 cm above the patient.

We use a 90° resectoscopic unipolar loop to cut the base of the polyp with a pure cutting current of 100 W. The end of the loop should be visualized all the time to avoid perforation. Movement should be controlled and directed toward the cervix. Bleeding can be coagulated with light application of the loop

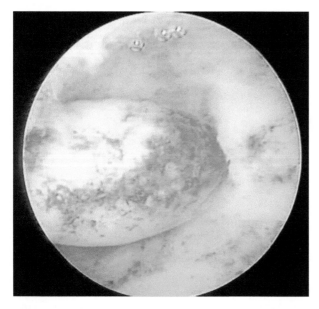

Figure 30.1 Endometrial polyp. (Courtesy of Togas Tulandi.)

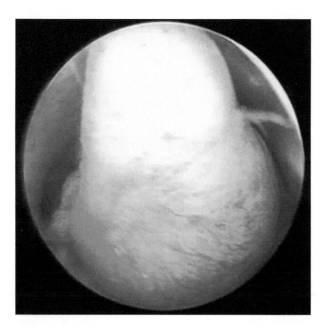

Figure 30.2 Large endometrial polyp. (Courtesy of Togas Tulandi.)

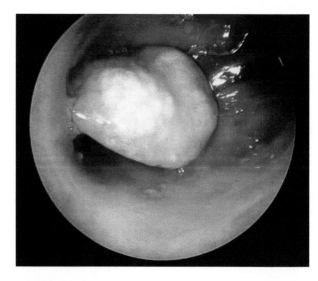

Figure 30.3 Submucous myoma, type 0.

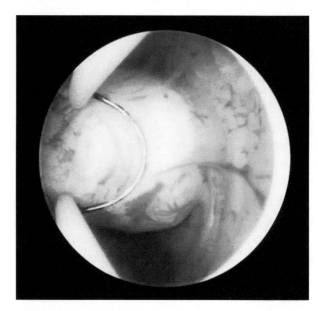

Figure 30.4 Submucous myoma, type 1.

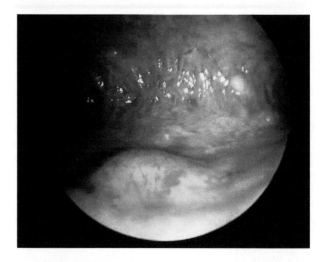

Figure 30.5 Submucous myoma, type 2.

electrode. In general, bleeding is minimal and does not require any treatment.

Hysteroscopic myomectomy

Hysteroscopic myomectomy is the treatment of choice for submucous myoma that is entirely (type 0) or mostly (type 1) located inside the uterine cavity. Fibroids that extend deep into the myometrium (type 2) can also be excised hysteroscopically using techniques such as uterine massage and dissection with a cold-knife electrode.

Removal of type 2 fibroids is more challenging, however. The operability depends on the size of the myoma (usually <5 cm) and the thickness of the remaining myometrium between the deep edge of the myoma and the outer surface of the uterus. Most authors set this safety margin at 0.5–1 cm. The risk of fluid overload or uterine perforation may lead to incomplete resection. The likelihood of achieving complete removal of type 2 fibroids is 50%.

We start the resection with anterior wall fibroids. This is to avoid air bubbles obscuring the operative field. The loop electrode is placed distal to the myoma and retracted toward the cervix. The large myoma is systematically cut with the loop until its pedicle is reached (Figure 30.6). We use a blend of currents, with 100 W for cutting and 50 W for coagulation.

Although incomplete resection of uterine fibroids is associated with failure of treatment and recurrent symptoms, there are several reports suggesting that residual tissue may undergo spontaneous regression, without the need for subsequent surgery.

COMPLICATIONS AND THEIR PREVENTION

- *Cervical lacerations* can occur from the tenaculum site. They are easily controlled by pressure applied with a sponge forceps. Rarely, a suture is needed. Tears can also result from difficult cervical dilatation, especially in postmenopausal/ nulliparous women or patients who previously received a GnRHa.
- The incidence of *uterine perforation* is estimated to be 0.4–1.6%. If perforation is suspected, laparoscopy should be performed to evaluate the integrity of the abdominal viscera. An intrauterine balloon is not recommended, as it might enlarge the tear or divert bleeding into the peritoneal cavity.
- *Fluid overload and electrolyte imbalance* are severe complications of operative hysteroscopy. Pulmonary and cerebral edema, coagulopathy, or

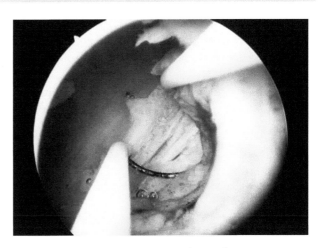

Figure 30.6 Type 2 myoma, resected to its base.

hyponatremia could develop. Fluid management is essential. Careful monitoring of the patient and administration of intravenous furosemide might be needed. One should abandon the procedure if the fluid deficit is more than 1000 ml (Chapter 36).

- *Incomplete removal.* The use of a preoperative GnRHa leads to a decrease in fibroid size and fluid loss during surgery, which facilitates complete removal of large fibroids. However, pretreatment with a GnRHa may render small myomas less visible and increases the probability of recurrence.
- *Bleeding.* Myometrial contraction is usually sufficient to control bleeding. However, in some patients, intravenous administration of uterotonic drugs or insertion of a Foley catheter balloon into the uterine cavity might be needed.
- *Postoperative uterine infection.* We use prophylactic antibiotics for hysteroscopic myomectomy.

SUGGESTED READING

- Nagele F, O'Connor H, Davies A, et al. 2500 outpatient diagnostic hysteroscopies. Obstet Gynecol 1996;88:87–92.
- Marsh FA, Rogerson LJ, Duffy SR. A randomised controlled trial comparing outpatient versus daycase endometrial polypectomy. BJOG 2006;113: 896–901.

- Varasteh NN, Neuwirth RS, Levin B, Keltz MD. Pregnancy rates after hysteroscopic polypectomy and myomectomy in infertile women. Obstet Gynecol 1999;94:168–71.
- Wamsteker K, Emanuel MH, de Kruif JH. Transcervical hysteroscopic resection of submucous fibroids for abnormal uterine bleeding: results regarding the degree of intramural extension. Obstet Gynecol 1993; 82:736–40.
- Murakami T, Tamura M, Ozawa Y, et al. Safe techniques in surgery for hysteroscopic myomectomy. J Obstet Gynaecol Res 2005;31:216–23.

31

Endometrial ablation

Roger Hart and Adam Magos

Endometrial ablation is designed to reduce excessive menstrual blood loss in women without uterine pathology, as an alternative to hysterectomy. With the advent of levonorgestrel-releasing intrauterine devices, the number of women undergoing surgical management of menorrhagia has diminished over time.

Today, there has been an increase in the use of second-generation endometrial ablation techniques. These techniques do not employ a hysteroscope, so they have the perceived benefit of a shorter learning curve. Surgeons should evaluate the endometrial cavity with either hysteroscopy or saline-infusion sonography before performing endometrial ablation.

FIRST-GENERATION TECHNIQUES

Transcervical endometrial resection (TCRE)

Hart and Magos in 1997 reported that, after 5 years, among women who had undergone the procedure of transcervical endometrial resection (TCRE), 26–40% were amenorrheic, 71–80% reported an improvement in the symptom of dysmenorrhea, and 79–97% were satisfied with their treatment. Ultimately, 9% of women underwent hysterectomy for the symptom of either pain or bleeding. However, even after 10 years, over 70% of women avoid hysterectomy.

Data derived from randomized controlled trials demonstrate that, compared with hysterectomy, TCRE is associated with a shorter operating time, fewer complications, less analgesic requirement, a faster resumption of normal activities, and greater cost–effectiveness. However, the satisfaction rate in women randomized to hysterectomy is slightly higher than in those randomized to endometrial resection.

Instrumentation and preoperative preparation

- Prior to surgery, it is essential to ensure that the patient has completed her family, that she has menorrhagia sufficient to warrant surgery and has exhausted medical management options, and that she understands the remote possibility of the procedure converting to a hysterectomy due to an unexpected complication.

- The use of either a gonadotropin-releasing hormone (GnRH) analogue or danazol prior to surgery, usually for 6 weeks, ensures that at the time of surgery the endometrium is thin. This pretreatment reduces operating time, intraoperative bleeding, and fluid absorption.

Procedure (Figures 31.1–31.5)

- TCRE is frequently performed under general anesthesia, although it may be performed with spinal or local anaesthesia (intra- and paracervical block and intrauterine injection of local anaesthesia in association with intravenous sedation). Most surgeons administer prophylactic antibiotics to limit postoperative febrile morbidity. The perineum and vagina are cleaned and the cervix is dilated to 10 mm.

- The equipment that is most frequently used consists of a 26 Fr continuous-flow passive-handle

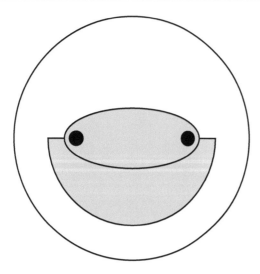

Figure 31.1 The upper posterior part of the endometrium is treated first.

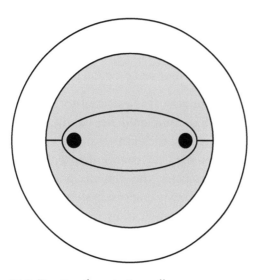

Figure 31.2 Treating the anterior wall.

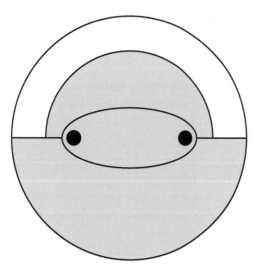

Figure 31.3 Completing ablation of the posterior wall.

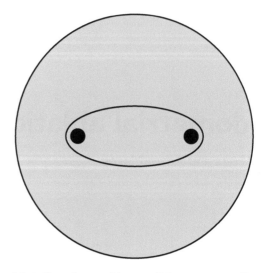

Figure 31.4 Completing ablation of the anterior wall.

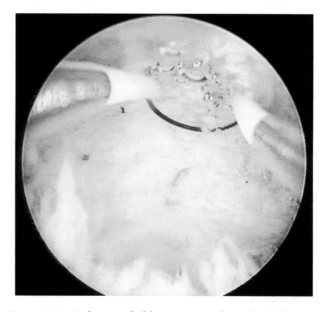

Figure 31.5 Endometrial ablation using a loop electrode.

resectoscope with a 4 mm fore–oblique hysteroscope and a 24 Fr cutting loop.

- To facilitate distention of the uterine cavity, a dedicated pump is employed that is able to control the flow rate and pressure of the distention fluid. The intrauterine pressure should be maintained between 80 and 120 mmHg during the operation. If the intrauterine pressure is insufficient, the view of the endometrial cavity becomes inadequate, whereas the use of excessive distention can precipitate complications related to fluid overload. To maintain continuous flow, and hence facilitate a clear operative field, a suction device is attached to the outflow of the resectoscope to maintain a negative pressure of about 50 mmHg. The negative pressure may be increased if the view is too cloudy, or decreased if the there is inadequate uterine distention prior to increasing the distention pressure.

- Resection of the endometrium is started with a blended monopolar cutting current at a power setting of 100–120 W. If submucous fibroids are present, these should be first resected with either a forward-angled cutting loop or a rollerball. The remainder of the uterine cavity is resected in a systematic manner, down to the internal os, with the conventional backward-pointing loop. The basic technique involves pushing the cutting loop out under direct vision and then, as soon as the loop is activated, drawing it in toward the sheath while applying pressure into the myometrium.

- The depth of resection is judged by the appearance of the circular muscle fibers; it is important not to cut too deeply, as this could potentially lead to bleeding and possible uterine perforation. The resected tissue chippings are pushed toward the fundus of the uterine cavity to enable visualization of the unresected part of the endometrial cavity, and are only removed at the end of the procedure, ideally using a flushing curette. This technique avoids the continual removal of the resectoscope from the uterine cavity, which increases the chance of cervical trauma and bleeding secondary to uterine cavity decompression. This is our preferred technique, but when the endometrium is thick, we resect the whole thickness of endometrium and remove the chippings with each pass of the resectoscope.

- The uterus is re-inspected at the end of the procedure to ensure that the resection is complete and that there are no bleeding vessels; the latter are usually easily controlled electrosurgically. If bleeding from the uterine cavity persists, a urinary catheter balloon inflated with 30 ml normal saline can be left inside the uterus for 4–6 hours to produce tamponade.

Distention media used for TCRE

The use of electricity to perform the resection requires the use of a nonconducting irrigating solution such as 1.5% glycine. It provides an excellent optical view and is nonhemolytic. Other less commonly used solutions include 5% dextrose in water, and a solution of 3% sorbitol, which is hyperosmolar (65–180 mosmol). Excessive absorption of this solution may lead to electrolyte disturbances, as well as glucostasis derangements. All electrolyte-free solutions can lead to dilutional hyponatremia and fluid overload.

Complications and their prevention

- *Excessive fluid absorption.* Excessive absorption of an electrolyte-free solution can be associated with hyponatremia and subsequently hemolysis. After absorbing 1 litre of glycine solution, the serum concentration of sodium will drop by approximately 10 mmol/l. In addition, a breakdown product of glycine is ammonia, which may produce an encephalopathy manifest by confusion, coma, and ultimately death (Chapter 36).

- *Uterine perforation and haemorrhage.* Potentially the most serious complication of TCRE is uterine perforation, with one national audit showing an overall risk of approximately 1.5–2.5%. Warning signs that uterine perforation has occurred include a sudden loss of uterine distention pressure and immediate loss of view. Unrecognized injury is a serious incident, as bowel or vascular injury may result from operating the resectoscope outside the uterus. The risk of infectious morbidity after surgery and intraoperative hemorrhage is approximately 1%.

- *Hematometra.* A late complication is the development of a hematometra due to an unresected area of endometrium at the fundus of the uterus or cervical stenosis. This is treated by a repeat resection and/or cervical dilatation, although caution needs to be exercised during entry into the uterine cavity to limit the risk of uterine perforation.

Rollerball endometrial ablation

This procedure relies on the same technique as that employed to treat the fundus of the uterus in TCRE. A ball electrode is moved across the endometrial surface, employing a blended cutting current to cause endometrial blanching and destruction.

The complications of this technique are similar to those of TCRE, although the risk of uterine perforation is less. The success rate of rollerball endometrial ablation is also similar to that of TCRE, with the disadvantages of absence of a histologic specimen.

Hysteroscopic laser ablation of fibroids

Laser ablation of the endometrium is now infrequently used. The equipment is expensive and must be regularly maintained. The results of endometrial ablation are similar to those with TCRE. Operative complications with laser endometrial ablation are similar to those of TCRE and occur in less than 5% of cases.

SECOND-GENERATION TECHNIQUES

These techniques do not require the same degree of technical expertise as the first-generation techniques. The majority do not require hysteroscopic control, and because they do not involve cutting, they have been marketed as 'safer' and 'easier'. The proof of safety has not yet been clearly demonstrated, although in certain situations where it is imperative to avoid fluid overload, such as in patients with significant cardiac disease, a second-generation technique may have advantages.

These techniques include nonhysteroscopic techniques such as balloon technology, microwave ablation, bipolar technology, diode lasers, monopolar energy, radiofrequency, cryotherapy, and photodynamic therapy. One technique employs hysteroscopic control using freely circulating hot water.

In a Cochrane review, overall the second-generation techniques appeared as effective as the first-generation techniques, although long-term follow-up data are still required for several newer techniques. Concerns that these nonhysteroscopic techniques may lead to an increased rate of unrecognized perforation and potential bowel injury were not confirmed by the review. However, the fact that these techniques are promoted as having the potential to be used by surgeons with limited operator skill is of concern, as is the frequent finding that several of the quoted studies reported a high degree of equipment failure with the second-generation procedures.

SUGGESTED READING

- Magos AL, Baumann R, Lockwood GM, Turnbull AC. Experience with the first 250 endometrial resections for menorrhagia. Lancet 1991;337: 1074–8.
- Overton C, Hargreaves J, Maresh M. A national survey of the complications of endometrial destruction for menstrual disorders: the MISTLETOE study. Br J Obstet Gynaecol 1997;104:1351–9.
- Hart R, Magos A. Endometrial ablation. Curr Opin Obstet Gynecol 1997;9:226–32.
- Garry R, Shelley-Jones D, Mooney P, Phillips G. Six hundred endometrial laser ablations. Obstet Gynecol 1995;85:24–9.
- Lethaby A, Hickey M, Garry R. Endometrial destruction techniques for heavy menstrual bleeding. Cochrane Database Syst Rev 2005;(4): CD001501.

32

Resection of uterine septum

Aarathi Cholkeri-Singh and Keith B Isaacson

Septate uterus occurs as a result of resorption failure of the septum that is formed when the two müllerian ducts fuse together. A complete septum may involve the upper two-thirds of the vagina, cervix, and uterine cavity, whereas a partial septum only involves the uterine cavity. Septate uterus has the highest rate of recurrent pregnancy losses and poor obstetric outcome, such as preterm labor, intrauterine fetal growth restriction, fetal malpresentation, and retained products of conception. Prior to the late 1980s, treatment of uterine septum was by a laparotomy approach.

Continuous-flow operative hysteroscopic metroplasty has replaced the traditional approach. With the hysteroscopic approach, the uterine musculature is not excised or traumatized. This allows a shorter recovery time and conception within 2 months after the procedure, and the patient can safely deliver vaginally. Similarly to abdominal metroplasty, term delivery rates after hysteroscopic metroplasty are approximately 80%, with a miscarriage rate of approximately 15%.

PREOPERATIVE IMAGING

To assess the shape of the uterine cavity, the most common imaging modality is hysterosalpingography (HSG) (Figure 32.1). However, HSG cannot assess the contour of the uterine fundus or differentiate between different types of uterine anomalies. Office hysteroscopy is another imaging modality, but like HSG, it cannot assess the uterine contour accurately. Combined diagnostic hysteroscopy and laparoscopy is the gold standard technique for diagnosing congenital müllerian anomalies.

Two-dimension (2D) transvaginal ultrasound is a good screening tool. Its sensitivity and specificity can be increased with saline-infused sonohysterography or 3D technology (Figure 32.2). The best nonsurgical technique for diagnosing and differentiating different types of uterine anomalies is magnetic resonance imaging (MRI). This is particularly useful to differentiate septate, bicornuate, or didelphys uterus.

PROCEDURE

The patient is placed in the dorsal lithotomy position. The perineum and vagina are prepared with sterile technique, and a catheter is used to empty the bladder. A speculum is placed, and the anterior lip of the cervix is grasped with a single-tooth tenaculum. If the cervix needs to be dilated, cervical dilators or dilute vasopressin are used. Otherwise, the hysteroscope is placed into the cervical canal using an operative sheath with a continuous-media-flow system and the speculum is removed.

When using a small operative hysteroscope, successful placement can be performed without a speculum or tenaculum by placing the hysteroscope into the vagina with an opened irrigating channel. The hysteroscope is inserted through the cervix and into the uterine cavity under direct visualization.

The optic lens used for visualization ranges from 12° to 30°. It is important to incise the septum in the midline and frequently obtain a panoramic view of the

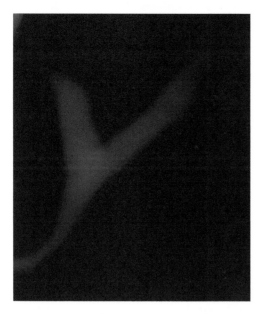

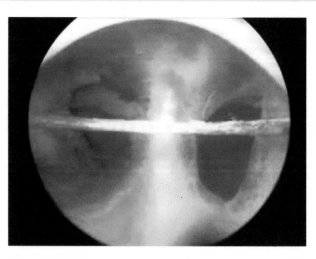

Figure 32.3 Hysterscopic image of uterine septum with loop accessory instrument for resection. (Photo courtesy of Dr. Najeeb M. Layyous, www. layyous.com).

Figure 32.1 Hysterosalpingogram image of uterine septum. (Photo courtesy of http://www.wegrijut.com/uterineanomalies/gallery.htm).

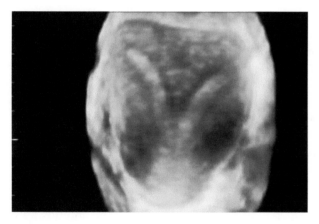

Figure 32.2 Three-dimensional image of uterine septum. (Photo courtesy of Dr. Najeeb M. Layyous, www.layyous.com).

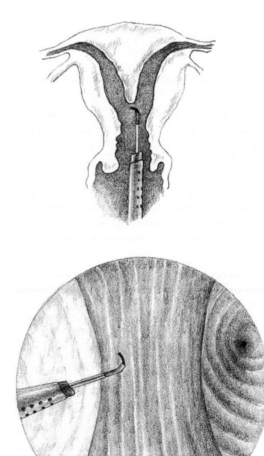

Figure 32.4 Division of the septum using a needle electrode.

cavity to reorient (Figures 32.3 and 32.4). The septum can be approached by two techniques. For a thin septum, the incision is in the midline, starting at the point closest to the cervix and continuing toward the fundus. For a thick septum, alternating incisions from side to side create a thinner septum that is subsequently treated as a thin septum. As the septum is incised, the anterior and posterior walls retract.

The septum is avascular. Bleeding usually occurs when the incision reaches the level of the myometrium at the fundus. The procedure is terminated at this point. Reproductive outcome is favorable, with a residual septum of <1 cm. Further septal resection is not recommended. Hysteroscopic septal resection can be performed with or without electrical or laser energy.

A complete septum involves the cervix. Some surgeons believe that resection of the cervical portion is associated with cervical incompetence. However, leaving the cervical portion of the septum might cause dystocia, preventing vaginal delivery. Our practice is to resect the cervical septum.

Instruments

Septal resection can be done using cold scissors (rigid or semirigid), laser fibers, a monopolar knife, loop electrodes and bipolar twizzle stick, or loop electrodes. The semirigid scissors are good for a thin septum and the rigid scissors for a thick septum. Laser and electrosurgery are quicker than scissors, but have the disadvantage of causing thermal injury to normal endometrial tissue. They are more dangerous than cold instruments should uterine perforation occur. A small operative sheath can be used for lasers, with the fiber being moved from side to side in the midline to incise the septum.

A thick septum is better incised with a loop electrode. Insertion of a resectoscope requires cervical dilatation up to 9 mm, and the use of electrolyte-free distention fluid. The loop is placed at a 90° angle along the septum and, with the cutting current, it is pressed up against the middle of the septum.

Additional imaging

To avoid incision into the myometrium, intraoperative use of other imaging modalities such as transabdominal ultrasound, intermittent fluorography, and laparoscopy are sometimes needed.

Post procedure

Postoperatively, the patient may experience a bloody discharge for up to 6 weeks. Hormonal treatment is not necessary; however, some physicians pretreat their patients with leuprolide to thin the endometrium. In this case, the patient should be treated with estrogen for 1 month, followed by progesterone in the last 5 days. Otherwise, the procedure is performed in the early proliferative phase. Typical follow-up with an HSG or office hysteroscopy to evaluate the success of the surgery is done within 2 months.

COMPLICATIONS AND THEIR PREVENTION

- Endometritis rarely occurs following operative hysteroscopy. The risk can be reduced by sterile preparation of the vaginal canal and perineum and by minimizing the number of insertions and reinsertions of the hysteroscope into the uterine cavity. Patients with a history of pelvic inflammatory disease should be given preoperative antibiotics.
- Bleeding rarely occurs. However, if the myometrium is disrupted, large venous sinuses can be encountered. To minimize intravasation, the intrauterine pressure should be reduced. Bleeding from small vessels can be controlled by laser or electrocautery. One can also perform bimanual compression of the uterus. An effective method is insertion of a Foley catheter into the uterine cavity, with the balloon being filled with 15–30 cm^3 of normal saline. The catheter is left in situ for a few hours to overnight.
- Intrauterine adhesion rarely occurs.
- Similarly to other hysteroscopic procedure, other possible complications are fluid overload and electrolyte imbalance, and uterine perforation (Chapter 36).

SUGGESTED READING

- Bacsko G. Uterine surgery by operative hysteroscopy. Eur J Obstet Gynecol Reprod Biol 1997;71:219–22.
- Homer HA, Li TC, Cooke ID. The septate uterus: a review of management and reproductive outcome. Fertil Steril 2000;73:1–14.
- Pabuccu R, Gomel V. Reproductive outcome after hysteroscopic metroplasty in women with septate uterus and otherwise unexplained infertility. Fertil Steril 2004;81:1675–8.
- Abu-Musa A, Chahine R, Aridi O, et al. Successful pregnancy outcome following Tompkins metroplasty done in early pregnancy. Hum Reprod 1998;13: 1387–8.

33

Transcervical tubal cannulation for treatment of proximal tubal occlusion

Spyros Papaioannou and John M Jafettas

Some 5–20% of hysterosalpingograms reveal proximal tubal occlusion (PTO). There are two types of proximal tubal occlusion. True occlusion can be due to salpingitis, endometriosis, or (rarely) congenital malformation. Another type is apparent proximal occlusion due to tubal spasm at the time of hysterosalpingography. Owing to the high incidence of false positives, a hysterosalpingographic finding of PTO must be followed by selective tubal catheterization. The cumulative pregnancy rate after tubal catheterization is 28% at 12-month follow-up. Approximately 20% of tubes cannot be catheterized; such patients are best treated by in vitro fertilization (IVF).

Selective tubal catheterization offers outpatient treatment and a safe procedure. Several transcervical tubal cannulation techniques have been described. The most commonly used are fluoroscopically guided selective salpingography and tubal catheterization and hysteroscopic tubal cannulation. The fluoroscopic procedure is beyond the scope of this chapter.

HYSTEROSCOPIC TUBAL CANNULATION

We use the Novy cornual cannulation catheter set (Cook UK, Letchworth, Hertfordshire, UK). It consists of an introducing catheter with an obturator, an inner catheter, and a wire guide.

The 5.5 Fr curved (55°) polyethylene introducing catheter is 40 cm long with a 3 cm clear tip. We can attach a plastic Y-shaped adapter with Luer-lock hub ends to the distal end of the introducing catheter. A detachable screwcap seals the straight arm of the adapter. This channel is used for irrigation or suction of the uterine cavity. The other arm of the Y-adapter is fitted with a 'stop-leak' Luer lock, which provides a tight seal around the inner catheter. A stainless steel obturator with an introducer allows one to adjust the shape of the distal catheter. The 3.0 Fr (2.5 Fr tip) translucent inner catheter is 55 cm long. The guidewire is 60 cm long and 0.46 mm in diameter. It is made of stainless steel and coated with a hydrophilic layer. It has a flexible blunt tip and a removable silicone safety cap at its distal end.

The spontaneous pregnancy rates following hysteroscopic tubal cannulation are 29–71.4%, and the ectopic pregnancy rates 3.6–5.9%.

PROCEDURE (FIGURES 33.1 AND 33.2)

We conduct the procedure in the follicular phase of the cycle. To exclude concomitant distal tubal disease, a laparoscopy is first performed. A second surgeon performs the hysteroscopy – ideally using a second light source and monitor.

Following identification of the tubal ostia, the surgeon inserts an introducing catheter with an obturator into the operating channel of the hysteroscope until its tip is visualized in the uterine cavity. A 30° lens is used. The obturator is then removed, and the end is sealed with a plastic cup or a syringe for chromotubation. The operator then introduces the inner catheter with the guidewire inserted.

Once visible at the tip of the introducing catheter, the guidewire leads the way. As the protruding

(a)

(b)

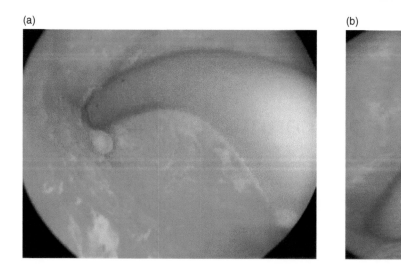

Figure 33.1 (a,b) Hysteroscopic tubal cannulation. (Courtesy of Gary Frishman.)

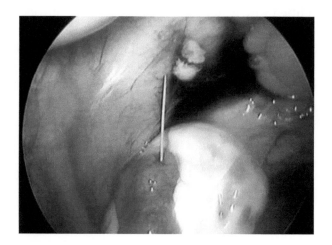

Figure 33.2 Laparoscopic view of transcervical tubal cannulation. (Courtesy of Gary Frishman.)

COMPLICATIONS AND THEIR PREVENTION

- The most common complication is tubal perforation. This occurs in up to 10% of cases. It is a minor complication that does not need any treatment.
- Vasovagal reaction can occur in 0.5% of cases.
- We administer prophylactic antibiotics and rarely encounter infection. Infection can occur in the presence of undiagnosed hydrosalpinges. In fact, a case of septic shock has been reported.
- Ectopic pregnancy has been reported in 3.6–5.9% of cases following hysteroscopic tubal cannulation.

CONTRAINDICATIONS

Women with distal tubal disease or previous tubal sterilization are not candidates for tubal catheterization. A previous tubal catheterization is not a contraindication, as repeat procedure has led to pregnancies. Tubal catheterization is not indicated for women who are undergoing IVF treatment.

SUGGESTED READING

- Papaioannou S. A hypothesis for the pathophysiology and natural history of proximal tubal blockage. Hum Reprod 2004;19:481–5.

guidewire lengthens, it becomes more flexible. The system is advanced through the uterotubal junction under laparoscopic control. The laparoscopist can facilitate cannulation by manipulating the tube to decrease the angle between the cornu and the isthmus. If resistance is felt, the inner catheter is advanced over the guidewire, which is then withdrawn. Tubal patency is evaluated by injecting a dilute solution of methylene blue into the inner catheter. If the fallopian tube is obstructed, the guidewire is reintroduced and gently pushed to overcome the obstruction. Patency is rechecked. The procedure is repeated on the opposite side.

- Honore GM, Holden AE, Schenker RS. Pathophysiology and management of proximal tubal blockage. Fertil Steril 1999;72:950–1.
- Papaioannou S, Afnan M, Girliny AJ, et al. The potential value of tubal perfusion pressures measured during selective salpingography in predicting fertility. Hum Reprod 2003;18:358–63.
- Novy MJ, Thurmond AS, Pathon P, Uchida BT, Rosch J. Diagnosis of cornual obstruction by transcervical fallopian tube cannulation. Fertil Steril 1988;50: 434–40.
- Papaioannou S, Afnan M, Girling AJ, et al. Long-term fertility prognosis following selective salpingography and tubal catheterization in women with proximal tubal blockage. Hum Reprod 2002;17: 2325–30.

34

Hysteroscopic tubal sterilization

Lynne Chapman and Adam Magos

Over more than a century, investigations have evolved in the search for an ideal method of female sterilization – a technique that can be done in an outpatient setting, without general anesthesia, that is simple, quick, easily learned, associated with few side-effects, and preferably reversible. Hysteroscopic sterilization has the potential to fulfill these criteria, but until recently has remained more of an ideal concept than a reality.

METHODS OF NONLAPAROSCOPIC STERILIZATION

Quinacrine

Quinacrine has been used for female sterilization for many years. However, there are concerns about its toxicity. In addition, it needs multiple applications, and there is a problem of confirming tubal occlusion. In a review of 2592 cases of quinacrine sterilization in Chile, there were 119 pregnancies, and the cumulative lifetime pregnancy rates per 100 women at 10 years varied from 5.2 to 6.9. Quinacrine sterilization is associated with low cost and can be performed by nonmedical personnel.

Ovabloc

Ovabloc (Fame Medical Products) is another old method of nonlaparoscopic sterilization (Figure 34.1). In a study of 392 women, the procedure could not be done in 13% of patients. Over 90% of patients retained the plug and two patients conceived. Twenty

women spontaneously expelled their plugs, and 10 had plugs removed due to side-effects.

Transcervical sterilization devices

Several intratubal ligation devices are available. The Essure System (Conceptus, Inc.) is the only one that is currently licensed for clinical use (Figure 34.2). Similar to Essure, another system that causes scarring and permanent tubal occlusion is the Intratubal Ligation Device (BioMedical Engineering Solutions, Inc.) (Figure 34.3).

The Complete TransCervical Sterilization System (Adiana, Inc.), on the other hand, combines controlled thermal damage of the endosalpinx and insertion of a biocompatible matrix within the tubal lumen (Figure 34.4). In contrast to other systems, no foreign body is left in the uterine cavity.

Other systems under investigation include the Ovion Eclipse (American Medical Systems), a nickel–titanium reversible tubal occlusion device (Berkeley Applied Science and Engineering), and a polytetrafluoroethylene tubal screw (Figure 34.5).

ESSURE SYSTEM

The Essure System (Figure 34.2) is an attractive alternative to laparoscopic sterilization and is being used and tested worldwide. Clinical trials have shown the method to be safe, acceptable, and effective. There is high patient acceptability, safety, and cost–benefit when compared with laparoscopic approaches.

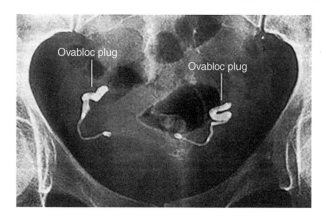

Figure 34.1 X-ray of Ovabloc in situ.

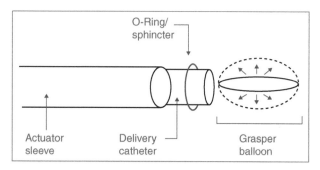

Figure 34.3 A diagram of the Intratubal Ligation Device. (After McClellan A. Slide presented at Clinical Update on Transcervical Sterilization, 8 December 2001, Baltimore.)

(a)

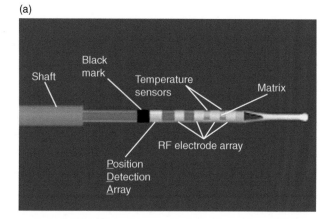

(b)

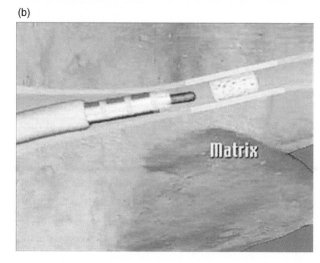

Figure 34.4 Complete TransCervical Sterilization System: (a) the coaxial automated catheter links to the radiofrequency generator; (b) a lesion is created, the catheter sheath retracts, a matrix is deposited, and the catheter is withdrawn.

(a)

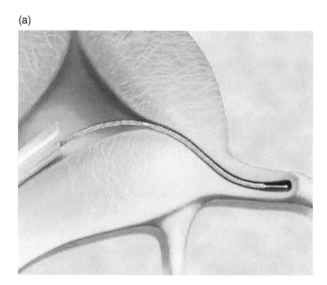

(b)

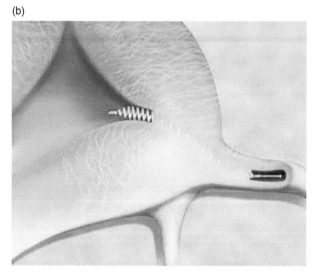

Figure 34.2 (a) Insertion of Essure. (b) Essure occluding the fallopian tube.

Essure is an expanding spring device (2 mm in diameter and 4 cm long) made of titanium, stainless steel, and nickel and containing Dacron fibers. It induces an inflammatory response and fibrosis of the

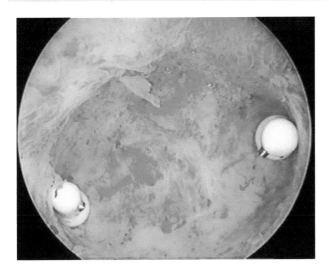

Figure 34.5 Tubal screws in situ.

intramural tubal lumen. The device can be inserted under ultrasound, fluoroscopic, or hysteroscopic guidance.

Initial studies have shown that bilateral placement is feasible in 81–95% of cases, and once in situ, it is effective in 99.8% of women. Placement of this system is operator-dependent. For example, in one study, all women who underwent laparoscopic sterilization had the procedure successfully completed, whereas the overall bilateral device placement rate for Essure was only 81%.

Procedure

The procedure is performed in the follicular phase of the cycle and under conscious sedation. In the lithotomy position, hysteroscopy is performed using a 5 mm hysteroscope with saline as the distention medium. The Essure device, placed at the tip of a disposable plastic handle, is inserted through the hysteroscope's 5 Fr working channel. After approaching the tubal ostium, the microinsert is placed in the intramural part of the tube, expanded so that between 3 and 12 loops of the spring remain visible, and detached from the handle.

The remaining catheter is then retrieved from the hysteroscope. The same procedure is repeated in the opposite tube.

COMPLICATIONS AND THEIR PREVENTION

- Apart from potential difficulties with bilateral placement, there is a delay in efficacy until sufficient tubal scarring has taken place.
- There is a possibility of nickel allergy.
- Besides pregnancy, there are other concerns with Essure. Hysteroscopic electrosurgery close to the device could present a risk. In addition, it might interfere with endometrial ablation using a loop or rollerball electrode.
- Patients might regret undergoing the procedure and wish to conceive with in vitro fertilization. The possible adverse effects on future pregnancy are unknown.

SUGGESTED READING

- Zipper J, Trujillo V. 25 years of quinacrine experience in Chile: review of 2,592 cases. In J Gynecol Obstet 2003;83:S23–9.
- Ubeda A, Labastida R, Dexeus S. Essure; a new device for hysteroscopic tubal sterilization in an outpatient setting. Fertil Steril 2004;82:196–9.
- Cooper JM, Carignan CS, Cher D, Kerin JF. Microinsert non-incisional hysteroscopic sterilization. Obstet Gynecol 2003;102:59–67.
- Duffy S, Marsh F, Rogerson L, et al. Female sterilization; a cohort controlled comparative study of Essure versus laparoscopic sterilization. BJOG 2005;112: 1522–8.
- Valle RF, Valdez J, Wright TC, Kenney M. Concomitant Essure tubal sterilization and Thermachoice endometrial ablation: feasibility and safety. Fertil Steril 2006; 86:152–8.

35

Anticipation and management of laparoscopic complications

Dan C Martin

The purpose of this chapter is to remind physicians of the possibility of damage that can occur related to laparoscopy and possible approaches to decrease it. Discussions of procedures and complications are given in the preceding chapters of this book.

Be prepared for complications and emergencies – they will occur. These might be related to the primary disease process, associated disease processes, healing process, patient positioning, preoperative care, intraoperative care, and postoperative care. Some complications, such as thromboembolism and infection, have specific preoperative prophylactic protocols. Others may be limited by appropriate education and experience. However, some complications may occur despite knowledge and experience.

Concepts of safety are frequently related to what authors assume to be effective and logical rather than evidence-based medicine. This is likely to continue to be a limitation as the number of patients required to perform an adequate blinded, randomized, prospective, controlled trial is significant – many of the major complications of laparoscopy occur at around or less than 1 in 1000 patients.

Although complications and errors will occur in medical care and surgery, our plan is to minimize the possibility, recognize the occurrence, and minimize the morbidity. This involves attention to equipment, personnel, the disease process, the healing process, and preoperative, intraoperative, and postoperative managements. Understanding anatomy and how it affects surgery is important. Knowledge of normal anatomy includes not only the uterus, tubes, ovaries, and their supporting structures but also the bladder, ureters, bowel, vessels, and lateral supporting tissue.

Education and team management are important in preparing for intraoperative care and for complications. Preoperative preparation, intraoperative technique, and postoperative surveillance are important parts of patient care. Surgeons should be comprehensive in all three areas. The suggestions and conclusions of this chapter may be controversial. Readers are encouraged to follow ongoing changes and development in the literature, as well as concepts, mechanisms, and clinical safety.

CULTURE OF SAFETY

As long as humans function in complex environments, errors will occur. The best that organizations can hope for is to manage error effectively, decrease the probability of errors, and minimize their consequences. Error is part of the human condition.

Training and education on inanimate objects, in the laboratory, and under video guidance has helped decrease the number of cases needed to pass the learning curve. Currently, a learning plateau occurs at 1–80 cases.

PREOPERATIVE CARE

History

Preoperative patient assessment and selection is needed to prepare the gynecologist and the patient for surgery. Laparoscopy for patients who have a history of bowel surgery requires considerations that are more complex than those for patients with no previous surgery undergoing tubal sterilization. Care to history and to physical examination may help to limit inappropriately chosen cases.

Medical history, current medications, and surgical history are essential. Certain medical problems, allergies, or reactions may change the need for preoperative management, evaluation, or stabilization. Surgical history may change the approach to surgery. Specifically questioning about appendectomy, tonsillectomy, laparoscopy, and cesarean section may reveal that patients did not consider these in a general question regarding surgery. In addition, some patients will forget certain operations that may be suggested only when examination of the abdomen reveals incisions that were not anticipated.

Since complications will be an anticipated part of any procedure, these need to be discussed with the patient. They should also be discussed with family members when this is reasonable. The risks, benefits, indications, alternatives, decreased sexuality, bleeding, blood transfusion, hysterectomy, paralysis, and death are subjects that I generally discuss for laparoscopic procedures.

Alternative treatment may include medical, radiologic, and other surgical management that may alter risks or benefits. Alternate possibilities that may occur during surgery and plans that may be needed during surgery are also considerations. Multiple plans may be needed. This is particularly true with multiple myomas, recurrent endometriosis, dermoids, and a history of significant adhesions. These can include decisions regarding when to stop surgery, when to proceed with an increased risk of hysterectomy and blood transfusion, or when to proceed to hysterectomy. Although infertility patients will generally desire preservation of the uterus, patients who have completed their childbearing and wish a complete operation may desire to proceed directly to hysterectomy if this is deemed necessary.

Prevention of thromboembolism

History, examination, and surgical plans may also suggest that thromboembolism prophylaxis is needed. This can include a combination of early mobilization, antiembolism stockings, intermittent pneumatic compression,

unfractionated heparin, low-molecular-weight heparin, and warfarin. Protocols for determining the specific prophylaxis are available from several sources. One version on the web is at http:// www.gp-training.net/ protocol/cardiovascular/ dvt.htm.

In addition, special attention to thromboembolism prophylaxis is given to women taking oral contraceptive pills (OCPs) and hormone replacement therapy (HRT). There may be no need to stop progesterone-only preparations. The risks of combined OCPs are more controversial. Considerations balance a small absolute excess risk in users against the risks of stopping the pill several weeks prior to surgery. The major risk is unplanned pregnancy, the effects of surgery and anesthesia on an unexpected pregnancy, and the risks of delayed surgery. The combined OCP can be continued without prophylaxis in women undergoing uncomplicated minor procedures. The risks require increased consideration of whether or not to stop the pill and whether to use antithrombosis prophylaxis in moderate-risk patients. HRT is often stopped several weeks prior to surgery, or antithrombosis prophylaxis can be used. Each case is considered individually in consultation with the patient.

For any surgery that is performed in a surgery center, the possibility of transfer to a hospital is anticipated. The surgeon must be prepared to admit the patients to an alternative hospital.

INTRAOPERATIVE CARE

Patient positioning

Position techniques can be specific for the stirrups and degree of table tilt used. Stirrup companies have videos and in-service material available with information on proper positioning. The degree of table tilt can be a problem if patients slide up the table. If shoulder supports are used, these need to be padded and adequate to stop the patient from sliding without damage.

Insertion techniques

There are proponents of open techniques, closed techniques, visual trocars, minilaparotomy, and others. Alternative site incisions and entrance sites for the trocar have also been suggested. Despite the multiple methods described for creating a pneumoperitoneum, there is no method that can claim to be superior to any other in all cases.

Most authors report on their favorite techniques without using blinded, randomized, prospective, controlled trials, and report these in series that are inadequate to draw conclusions. They are unlikely to publish data that showed that they had bad experiences. If the complication rate is 1–2 per 1000, then a randomized prospective study might require 2500 patients in each arm to detect a statistically significant difference. This would be an expensive and difficult study. No matter how much technical innovation occurs, the promises of safety need to be balanced by good judgment and proper technique. A separate concern is that changing from an accustomed technique to a new technique may increase complications and risks.

Insertion techniques such as the Hasson approach have been suggested as ways to avoid bowel and vascular injury. However, some data suggest that this approach may increase the risk to the bowel and does not completely avoid vascular damage. Although the proponents suggest that the increase in bowel damage is related to patient's selection, my experience is that there is an increase in bowel damage related to trying to enter the abdomen through a small incision. My impression is that small incisions are not good for palpation and recognition of the bowel or for limiting bowel injury. If one wishes to avoid injury using laparotomy, then it is important to ensure that the incision is large enough that the bowel can be palpated. Open laparoscopy also presents a disadvantage in terms of leaking of gas and difficulty in entrance.

Injury can occur at both needle insertion and trocar insertion (Figures 35.1–35.4). After insertion, one should examine the area directly beneath the trocar, above the insertion site, and below the insertion site. The anatomy should be normal and there should be no evidence of bowel damage, including abnormal fluid. If there is abnormal anatomy, the position of the bowel should be clarified with respect to the insertion site. Insertions have been made with through-and-through incision to the bowel. In some of these circumstances, the bowel perforation was not recognized until the end of the case. If there is any suggestion of bowel perforation, sufficient additional probes should be placed to allow careful examination of both sides of

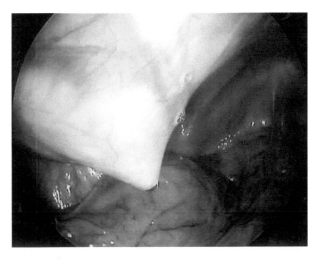

Figure 35.1 The tip of the trocar is lateral to the inferior epigastric vessels.

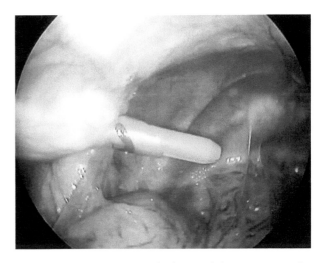

Figure 35.2 The trocar is pushed toward the anterior midline of the pelvis.

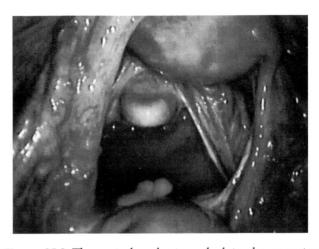

Figure 35.3 The vaginal probe is pushed in the posterior vaginal fornix.

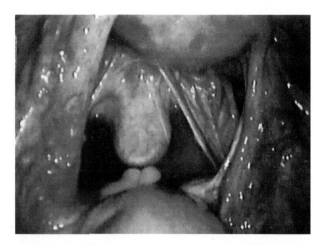

Figure 35.4 The vaginal probe is pushed into the middle of the posterior vagina near the rectal reflection.

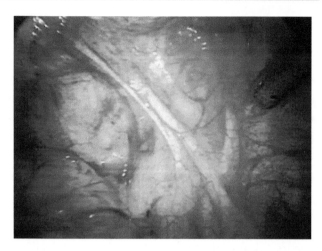

Figure 35.5 The ureter is adjacent to the uterosacral ligament in the picture. The ureteral position in the broad ligament is variable.

the length of the bowel. Intraoperative recognition and repair can avoid the increased morbidity of delayed diagnosis.

Factors that appear to increase bowel injuries are a history of laparotomy, very obese or very thin patients, multiple insertion techniques of the various instruments, performing enterolysis, and performing adhesiolysis. Although some authors suggest that bowel preparation is useful, others suggest that this does not change the course. Recent publications and general surgery literature suggest a decreased use of bowel preparation.

Anatomy

The anatomy of the pelvis should be clarified at the beginning, during, and at the end of the procedure. Attention to the various organs may help to decrease the chance of injury. Particular attention should be paid to the location of the ureter (Figure 35.5), lateral vessels, rectosigmoid colon, and bladder. Any surgery in the deep pouch of Douglas may be on or near the bowel. One should plan to operate in the anterior midline. The anterior space helps to avoid the bowel, and a midline position helps to avoid the lateral vessels and ureter.

Bladder

Full-thickness bladder injury may have an entrance and exit. If an exit hole is found, one should be certain of the entrance site – use methylene blue or similar dye (a volume of 250 cm^3 may be

needed to demonstrate a leak). Foley catheter drainage for 7 to 10 days, followed by a cystogram, may be sufficient.

Vascular

Although vascular injury is uncommon, it can be devastating and associated with high morbidity and mortality. This could be due to needle insertion, trocar insertion, or incisions into the vessels.

Brisk bleeding suggests major vessel damage. Unless one is trained to repair vascular injury by laparoscopy, the best decision is to consult a vascular surgeon. He or she will repair the vessels (usually by laparotomy). If a hematoma is noted in the retroperitoneal area or bleeding is from an unseen site, this needs ongoing observation and/or surgery for clarification. Sonograms can be used to monitor the growth of a hematoma if it is appear to be stable at the time of laparoscopy. However, if stability is not clear, open surgery may be the better course.

Pneumothorax

Although rare pneumothorax is frequently attributed to diaphragmatic defects. Low insufflation pressures and observation by the anesthesiologist may help recognize the problem at low volume levels. If a pneumothorax occurs, corrective action is needed. This is generally recognized by the anesthesia team, but the gynecologist needs to be ready to deflate the abdomen in order to help provide supportive care.

Lysis of adhesions

Lysis of adhesions can be associated with increased complications. Intermittent reappraisal of normal and abnormal anatomy is needed during this process. Traction using bowel surfaces is avoided, as tension tears can occur in the bowel. Lysis of adhesions between vascular areas and bowel surfaces can increase the chance of damage to either structure (Figure 35.6).

Electrosurgery

Electrosurgical safety improves by understanding the basics of equipment, tissue effects, zones of injury, and types of injury. I suggest the use of nonmodulated (cutting) current unless modulated (coagulation) current is needed, using arcing to control the depth of penetration when there is slow bleeding and attempting to force the path of least resistance to less vital organs. The path of least resistance can be forced by coagulating an adhesion from the bowel to the uterus at its midpoint first, and then closer to the uterus. Cutting can then be at the closer edge of the uterus.

Electrodes are activated only when fully in the field of vision, and tension is avoided on the operating electrode while cutting adhesions. Correction on an adhesion can be performed with a separate instrument.

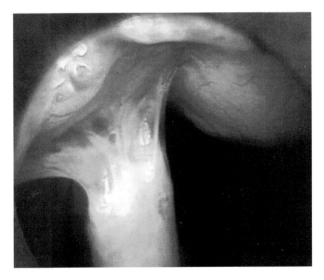

Figure 35.6 The initial dissection plane in this case had adequate separation of the bowel muscularis from the anterior wall. However, as dissection proceeded, the muscularis was noted immediately adjacent to the fascia, and further lysis was avoided.

Rigid electrosurgical probes do not waver as much as nonrigid probes, and may be safer. When organs are mobile, one should operate in the anterior midline of the pelvis in order to avoid electrosurgical damage to the lateral sidewalls, lateral vessels, ureter, and bowel.

Decreasing postoperative pain

A method to decrease postoperative pain and to increase the chance of recognizing complications is to instill 1–2 liters of Ringer's lactate at the end of a procedure. This will decrease the frequency of shoulder pain on sitting or standing. However, it is not likely to decrease the pain that is present when lying. That pain is related to diaphragmatic irritation occurring during surgery. Ringer's lactate is used, since saline is a peritoneal irritant. It has 40 mEq of lactate per liter, which approximates the buffering capacity of serum and avoids some of the problems of saline. Adept® is an alternative approved for adhesion prophylaxis in 2006. Adept® also uses lactate as the buffer.

POSTOPERATIVE CARE

Be prepared to transfer to hospital from a surgery center and be prepared to admit if the surgery is in the hospital. The laparoscopic surgeon should be aware of the risk of bowel injury and the grave consequences of delayed diagnosis. Immediate repair can decrease longterm complications and morbidity. A high index of suspicion of undiagnosed bowel injury should be raised in patients who do not improve steadily. This suspicion may improve recognition, but may also result in unnecessary laparotomies in patients with borderline findings.

Although patients generally do not feel well after surgery, they should improve progressively. This is particularly important when the surgery was in the vicinity of the bowel. Bowel perforation can present with subtle signs and symptoms and postoperative bowel management is complicated by the finding that normal signs expected in a bowel perforation are frequently not present. Many patients return to the emergency room a few days after discharge. They may have normal white blood cell count and temperature, no rebound, no rigidity, and tenderness only in the area of the incision – but this would be normal for surgery. A flat and upright abdomen for free air has a low sensitivity, and may pick up <70% of perforations. Even worse is the specificity of the finding of free air, which can be <1%. Although computed tomography (CT) can be used for perforation associated with inflammation, early perforation can still be missed. A Renografin® enema has been used to demonstrate rectal perforation missed by CT imaging. Early laparoscopy or laparotomy may miss a small perforation that will become larger due to ulceration.

Patients who do not void generally have short-term bladder retention that can be treated expectantly. However, they have to be investigated for the possibility of bladder perforation. Be careful to clarify postoperative coverage when you are not going to be available. When you are covering for another physician, evaluate more carefully than usual.

SUGGESTED READING

- Borten M, Freidman EA. Laparoscopic Complications: Prevention and Management. Philadelphia: BC Decker, 1986.
- Clements RV. Safe Practice in Obstetrics and Gynecology: a Medico-Legal Handbook. New York: Churchhill Livingston, 1994.
- Helmreich RL, Merritt AC. Culture at Work in Aviation and Medicine: National, Organizational and Professional Influences. Burlington, VT: Ashgate, 1998.
- Isaacson K. Complications of Gynecologic Endoscopic Surgery. Philadelphia: WB Saunders, 2006.
- Shapiro MJ, Morey JC, Small SD, et al. Simulation based teamwork training for emergency department staff: does it improve clinical team performance when added to an existing didactic teamwork curriculum? Qual Saf Health Care 2004;13:417–21.

36

Prevention, management, and legal aspects of hysteroscopic complications

Danielle E Luciano and Anthony A Luciano

Hysteroscopy is extremely useful in the evaluation and management of abnormal uterine bleeding, recurrent abortions, or uterine anomalies. Although rare (1–3%), complications occur more often with operative than with diagnostic hysteroscopy. The procedures commonly associated with complications are resection of uterine septum and lysis of uterine synechia, followed by removal of uterine fibroids and polyps.

CERVICAL LACERATION

Some of the frequent hysteroscopic complications are related to cervical dilatation, including cervical tears and creation of a false passage. They tend to occur in women with nulliparity, menopause, prior cervical surgery, and/or acutely ante- or retroverted uteri. In women at risk for cervical stenosis, preoperative cervical dilatation with laminaria or cervical softening with misoprostol should be considered. The vaginal administration of misoprostol, 400 µg 12 and 24 hours before surgery makes the cervix soft and easy to dilate, reducing the risk of laceration or of creating a false passage.

UTERINE PERFORATION

Uterine perforation occurs in approximately 1.5% of cases and accounts for approximately 30% of all hysteroscopic complications. The predisposing factors are similar to those of cervical laceration; as well as in patients with previous cone biopsy, or treated with a gonadotropin-releasing hormone (GnRH) agonist. The use of laminaria or misoprostol might decrease this complication. In patients at risk, preoperative assessment of the uterus by transvaginal ultrasound is helpful. Knowing the angle and the depth of the uterine cavity allows the operator to direct and choose the depth of dilator insertion.

Perforation is recognized by advancement of the dilator beyond the confines of the uterus, by hysteroscopic visualization of the perforation, and by a sudden large fluid deficit. At this point, the hysteroscopy should be stopped and the patient must be monitored for bleeding, which may occur vaginally, intraperitoneally or both. Examination of the abdomen by either pelvic ultrasound or laparoscopy is warranted, especially where there is significant vaginal bleeding. If intraperitoneal bleeding is suspected, laparoscopic exploration should be done (Figure 36.1). Laparoscopy also allows coagulation of the bleeding vessels and suturing of the perforation. The hysteroscopy can be resumed, completing the procedure. Otherwise, the patient should be rescheduled for the procedure at a later date, with preoperative cervical ripening agents and continuous laparoscopic monitoring.

DISTENTION MEDIA-RELATED COMPLICATIONS

Dextran 70

Problems associated with different distention media account for 10% of hysteroscopic complications and

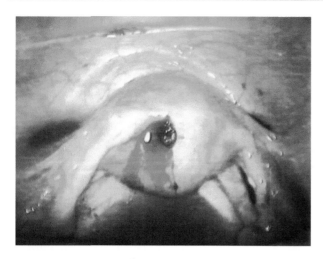

Figure 36.1 Uterine perforation.

are related to the type of medium used. The only currently available high-viscosity distention medium is Dextran 70 (Hyskon), a potent plasma expander. Intravenous infusion of $100\,cm^3$ of Hyskon increases the plasma volume by $860\,cm^3$.

Major complications associated with Hyskon intravasation include pulmonary edema, coagulopathies, and allergic reactions, from mild skin rashes to anaphylactic shock. The risk of pulmonary edema increases with fluid deficits >250 cm³ and with procedures lasting over 45 minutes. Anaphylaxis is seen in 1 in 1500 to 1 in 300 000 cases. In addition, excessive absorption of Dextran 70 can prolong bleeding time. It is rarely clinically relevant and is self-limiting. For these reasons, and because of its stickiness (which damages hysteroscopes), Hyskon is now rarely used.

Isotonic and hypotonic solutions

Ringer's lactate and normal saline are isotonic, electrolyte-containing media, and cannot be used with monopolar electrosurgery. This type of electrosurgery requires electrolyte-free solutions such as glycine 1.5%, a mixture of sorbitol 3% and mannitol 0.54%, or mannitol 5%. Isotonic solutions, such as mannitol 5%, are less likely to cause hypo-osmolality, but can also cause hypervolemia and hyponatremia.

- Excess intravasation of electrolyte fluids is associated with pulmonary edema, congestive heart failure, and hyperchloremic acidosis. Recognition of a large fluid deficit in conjunction with difficult

ventilation or auscultory signs of pulmonary edema are signs of fluid overload and necessitate cessation of the procedure, treatment with furosemide, and strict monitoring of the patient's input and output. Hyperchloremic acidosis is associated with impaired myocardial contractions, increased risk of ventricular fibrillation, tachycardia, and hypertension. Treatment for acidosis is sodium bicarbonate solution, furosemide, and oxygen.

- Electrolyte-free solutions metabolize into free water, which crosses into the intracellular and extracellular spaces, leading to hyponatremia in addition to hypervolemia. With each liter of hypotonic electrolyte-free solution that is absorbed, the serum sodium levels decrease by approximately 10 mmol. Symptoms of hyponatremia correlate and progress with decreasing serum sodium levels, as summarized in Table 36.1. Excess glycine or leucine absorption is also associated with an increase in serum ammonia levels, causing muscle aches, visual disturbances, and encephalopathy. In addition to treatment of hyponatremia, L-arginine administration may be effective.

The above complications could be avoided by strict monitoring of intake and output of the

Table 36.1 Symptoms of hyponatremia

Serum sodium (mmol/l)	Symptoms
130–135	Apprehension, disorientation, irritability, twitching, nausea/vomiting, shortness of breath
125–130	Pulmonary edema, moist skin, polyuria
120–125	Hypotension, bradycardia, cyanosis, mental status changes
115–120	Encephalopathy, congestive heart failure, lethargy, confusion, convulsions
<115	Brainstem herniation, respiratory arrest, coma, death

distending media and serum electrolyte levels. With fluid deficits of 500–1000 cm^3, blood for electrolyte measurement should be drawn immediately and furosemide should be administered. A Foley catheter is placed for accurate urinary output measurement. The procedure should be terminated immediately when the fluid deficit is 1500 cm^3. Treatment of hyponatremia is best done slowly, correcting serum sodium with intensive monitoring of patient input and output. Severe hyponatremia should be treated in consultation with an intensivist with central venous pressure (CVP) monitoring, diuretics, hypertonic saline, and fluid restriction.

- Early recognition of fluid deficit leads to prompt measures and avoidance of serious complications. Vigilant fluid monitoring is mandatory, and can be facilitated by the use of automated monitoring machines. For those who are using manual fluid monitoring, it is important to note that commercial intravenous solution bags can contain 5–10% more fluid than the bag indicates; for example a 3000 cm^3 bag can contain 300 cm^3 excess fluid.
- Fluid intravasation is enhanced by increased intrauterine pressure, prolonged surgical time, and cutting into open vascular channels, as with deep myometrial resection and large vascular fibroids. The possible hypervolemic complications can be minimized by keeping the intrauterine pressure at or below the mean arterial pressure, by avoiding cutting deep into the myometrium, by avoiding traumatic cervical dilatation, by avoiding the Trendelenberg position, and by operating quickly and efficiently. Some authors have suggested that preoperative use of GnRH agonists or intracervical injection of vasopressin may decrease fluid absorption.

HEMORRHAGE

Excessive intraoperative bleeding accounts for 1% of hysteroscopic complications and is most often associated with cervical injury or uterine perforation. Treatment involves suturing the laceration, followed by intrauterine balloon placement if needed. Rarely, bleeding cannot be controlled with these techniques. Early recognition and treatment can decrease serious complications. Patients should be counseled accordingly at the preoperative appointment.

INFECTION

- Endometritis is a rare complication of hysteroscopy, occurring in less than 1% of procedures. Most patients respond to oral antibiotics and rarely require hospitalization.
- Urinary tract infections and pelvic inflammatory disease are also rare complications.

The American College of Obstetrics and Gynecology does not recommend antibiotic prophylaxis for hysteroscopy, except in high-risk patients with a history of pelvic inflammatory disease, possible residual necrotic tissue from previous suction curettage, or intrauterine adhesions and endometritis. In these patients, we use doxycycline preoperatively. To prevent systemic herpes complications, hysteroscopy procedures should not be performed on women with active genital herpes lesions.

GAS OR AIR EMBOLISM

- Gas or air embolism is extremely rare (<0.05%) of hysteroscopic complications but is potentially fatal. Entry of carbon dioxide (CO_2) into the venous circulation is common when CO_2 is used as the distending medium. It is readily soluble in blood. However, when CO_2 insufflation is prolonged, gas embolism may occur, with dire consequences. Therefore, CO_2 should not be used in operative procedures.
- Air embolism is more common and more dangerous than CO_2 embolism, because 70% of air is nitrogen, which is insoluble in blood. It can occur via the tubing transporting distention fluid. This tubing should be purged. In addition, multiple insertions and reinsertions of cervical dilators or the hysteroscope can act as pistons that entrain air under pressure into the uterine cavity. Further, vigorous manipulations to overcome cervical stenosis can lead to formation of a false passage. The use of the Trendelenberg position promotes open access of air into the vascular tree.

The first and most common symptom of air embolism is a decrease in end-tidal CO_2. In this situation, a possible air embolism should be suspected and the procedure should be stopped. The chain of events that follows include hypotension, cardiac arrhythmia, mill-wheel murmur, and finally death. Prevention of this rare but life-threatening complication includes avoidance of the Trendelenberg position, monitoring and keeping the intrauterine pressure at or below the mean arterial pressure, flushing the fluid lines, gentle cervical dilatation, reducing instrument exchanges, and close monitoring of end-tidal CO_2. Treatment involves immediate discontinuation of the procedure, turning the patient to the left lateral decubitus position, and assisting ventilation with 100% oxygen.

LATE-ONSET COMPLICATIONS

Delayed complications of hysteroscopy are uncommon. They include hematometra, pregnancy complications, and delayed diagnosis of endometrial carcinoma.

- Hematometra is uncommon. It occurs with excessive scarring and narrowing of the endometrial cavity, usually following endometrial ablation/resection or removal of large submucosal myomas. Symptoms include cyclic or chronic lower abdominal pain in premenopausal females or postmenopausal females on hormone replacement. Treatment consists of cervical dilatation and evacuation of the uterine contents. In women with previous tubal sterilization, hematosalpinx can develop, and occasionally they may require unilateral or bilateral salpingectomy.
- Pregnancies after uterine ablation or resection are uncommon (<1%). Complications of this type of pregnancy include placenta accreta/ increta, intrauterine growth restriction, and preterm labor. Patients should be advised about the possibility of pregnancy after endometrial ablation and its possible risks.
- Uterine rupture/dehiscence has been reported following adhesiolysis, myoma resection, septolysis, and uterine perforations.
- Delayed diagnosis of endometrial carcinoma is rare. It is paramount to perform an endometrial

sampling before or during an endometrial ablation, especially in women at risk for endometrial carcinoma.
- Another potential risk of hysteroscopy is dissemination of endometrial cancer cells into the fallopian tube and the peritoneal cavity cells.

Table 36.2 Patient preparation to minimize hysteroscopy complications

Preoperative

- Patient history: need for cervical ripening agents (laminaria or misoprostol) or gonadotropin-releasing hormone agonist
- Comprehensive gynecologic evaluation: pelvic examination, imaging studies.
    - Vaginal ultrasound to determine the attitude and length of uterus facilitates cervical dilatation and may prevent perforation
- Laboratory measurements: blood count, baseline serum electrolytes, kidney function
- Informed consent: risks, benefits, expectations

Intraoperative

- Position patient flat or head-up. Avoid Trendelenberg position
- Purge all fluid lines of room air
- Gentle cervical dilatation to avoid creating false passages or perforating the uterus
    - Remember the distance from the cervix to the fundus measured by ultrasound
- Use continuous-flow instillation at the lowest possible pressure
- Use automated fluid management systems, monitoring fluid deficit and checking electrolytes as needed
- Work efficiently and keep the length of the procedure under 60 minutes
- Monitor cardiovascular parameters and remind the anesthesiologist of potential embolism
- Know when to abort the procedure, with evidence of rapid fluid absorption or blood loss

MINIMIZING COMPLICATIONS

Complications and adverse legal consequences of hysteroscopy mishaps can be minimized with adequate surgical training, proper patient selection, and early recognition and intervention of potential complications. As outlined in Table 36.2, recognizing the patient at risk for hysteroscopic complications is an essential part of the preoperative evaluation and proper management. The intraoperative preparation of the patient (including positioning on the table), conduct of the procedure, and monitoring of fluids and electrolytes assure that complications are averted or at least quickly recognized and appropriately treated. A knowledgeable surgical team is extremely important – from the anesthesiologist, who needs to be aware of signs and symptoms of air embolism and fluid overload, to the circulating and scrub nurses, who must be trained to handle hysteroscopic instruments and fluid monitoring.

SUGGESTED READING

- Aydeniz B, Gruber IV, Schauf B, et al. A multi-center survey of complications associated with 21,676 operative hysteroscopies. Eur J Obstet Gynecol Reprod Biol 2002;104:160–4.
- Grove JJ, Shinaman RC, Drover DR. Noncardiogenic pulmonary edema and venous air embolus as complications of operative hysteroscopy. J Clin Anesth 2004; 16:48–50.

Index

Page numbers in *italic* denote material in Figures or Tables.